Dr Jo's Serenity Prayer for Travelers:

God, grant me the wisdom to plan well for things I can control;
to retain patience, perspective, and a backup plan
when things I can't control go awry;
and the ability to laugh when nothing else works.

How to Stay Healthy & Fit on the Road

Joanne V. Lichten, PhD, RD

(aka Dr. Jo)

Nutrifit Publishing

How to Stay Healthy & Fit on the Road
Joanne V. Lichten, PhD, RD

Published by:
Nutrifit Publishing
PO Box 690452
Houston, TX 77269-0452
(281) 955-5326
(888) 431-5326
Email: DrJo@DrJo.com
www.DrJo.com

Printed in the USA

Publisher's Cataloging in Publication data:
Lichten, Joanne V.
How to Stay Healthy & Fit on the Road
(The ultimate health guide for the 44 million business and
93 million recreational travelers. Tips on defensive dining
on the road, fitting in exercise, getting a good night's
sleep, recovering from jet lag, and managing stress.)
208 pages

ISBN: 1-880347-53-9: $9.95 (pbk)

Cover design by Theresa Southwell

This book is dedicated to my daughter, Alexandra, who understands my need to travel and to my husband, Lorin, who is a pretty good "mommy" in my absence.

Many thanks to Lorin, Alexandra, and my Dad who spent many hours reading my book and offering suggestions.

I'd like to also express my appreciation to Christy Craig for her editorial assistance and Theresa Southwell for her creative cover design and interior illustrations.

Table of Contents

Continued on Next Page

Table of Contents

(continued)

Dear Fellow Traveler:

According to the Travel Industry Association of America, there are 44 million business travelers and 93 million recreational travelers. What all of us have in common is leaving - leaving the comfort of familiar surroundings for the uncertainty and excitement of what lies beyond the next bend.

If you're a business traveler, you may have heard people comment about all the fun and freedom you must be experiencing. This is hardly the emotion that most of us feel when we hit the road. Our travel is not our "raison d'être," but rather just the cost of doing business. When we compound work and family commitments with hectic, unpredictable travel schedules, drives in unfamiliar cities, a different hotel room every night, and the monotony and loneliness of eating in restaurants, we often impact our health negatively. It shows in unwanted weight gain, insomnia, and low energy levels.

Many recreational travelers (as a badge of honor) characterize their vacations in terms of weight gained. Returning more fatigued than when they left, they'll say "I need another vacation to recover from this one." Leisure travel need not be so exhausting.

It is my hope that this book will help make you healthier, happier, and most of all serves to recharge your batteries.

Dr Jo

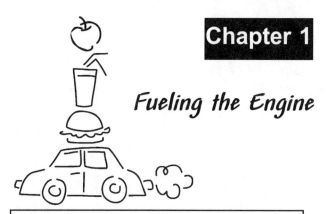

Chapter 1

Fueling the Engine

In This Chapter:
▶Start Your Engines
▶Defensive Dining on the Road
▶Meals on Wheels - healthy, packable foods
▶*Dr Jo's Eat Out & Lose Weight Plan*

Every engine needs the proper mix of high octane fuel, fluids, and additives to run at peak performance and our bodies
are no different. Unfortunately, we are more likely to obey
our car's recommended maintenance schedule than we are
to follow general healthy eating guidelines – and it shows.
More than 50% of all Americans are currently overweight
or obese. Topping off the fuel tank seems to be even more
prevalent amongst travelers since we eat out more often. In
addition, we're more likely to veer off our regular eating
schedule and indulge in fewer nutrition-packed foods. No
wonder we grow "spare tires" and feel sluggish when we
spend too much time on the road. But have no fear, it's easy
to eat healthy (and not feel deprived) when we follow a few
guidelines.

Start Your Engines

▶ **Fill Up Regularly.** It takes roughly five hours to digest a meal and absorb the nutrients. If we eat more than we need during that five hour period, the extra calories go into our "holding tanks." Some of us eat just once or twice a day and expect those holding tanks to provide us with the energy we need throughout the rest of the day. Although a small amount of energy is stored in our liver and muscles (in the form of glycogen) that is released quite easily, most of the energy is reserved in our holding tank called fat! And if fat cells could be broken down easily to provide us with energy – we'd all be skinny! Stop feeding your holding tank. Instead, eat regularly throughout the day. Sure you can still skimp at one meal when you know the next meal might be a bit heavier, but don't cut out the meal entirely!

- **Jumpstart your engine.** Why do you think they call the first meal of the day "break-fast"? Because it literally breaks the evening's fast. Breakfast gives us the energy we need to perform at our best and helps to jumpstart our metabolism. Have you ever skipped breakfast so you could enjoy the calories later in the day? Sounds like a good idea. However, it doesn't work that way. Breakfast eaters (because of the boost in the metabolism it causes) tend to be leaner than those who skip. In weight loss studies, breakfast skippers who began eating breakfast lost more weight than those who continued to skip.

- **Add fuel every five waking hours.** Skipping meals or delaying a meal tends to lead to overeating at the next meal. Remember that holding tank?

- **Take the edge off.** Since we can't always control our schedule, keep some healthy snacks with you. They'll always be late meetings, traffic jams, and cancelled flights, but at least you can be prepared.

▶ **Check Your Fluid Level.** Did you know that the human body is made up of 60% water? No wonder that even being slightly dehydrated can zap our energy. How do you know if your fluid level is low? Check your urine. If it's dark (it should be clear), you're not drinking enough!

- **Drink 6-8 glasses of water a day.** Thirst is often misinterpreted as hunger, so keep a bottle of water with you at all times. In restaurants, ask for a pitcher of water while you're waiting for your meal.

- **Limit your caffeinated beverages.** It doesn't appear to be harmful to have a cup or two of coffee (or other caffeinated beverages) to get you going in the morning. But caffeine is a diuretic that drains precious fluid from your body. It can also prevent you from relaxing and falling asleep at night (there's more on this in the *Snooze Control* chapter). Have you ever slept in on the weekend and woken up with a headache? Regular caffeine users find that skipping the usual "dose" of caffeine can bring on the wicked headache of caffeine withdrawal. If you want to cut back, it's best back off the caffeine slowly to avoid the headaches.

- **Watch the alcohol.** Are you enjoying a glass or two because you heard it was healthy for your heart? These benefits do not come without risks or calories. Risks such as alcohol addiction and car accidents are well known, however, alcohol consumption is also linked to increased triglycerides, blood pressure, and insomnia. While an occasional glass or two a day can be worked into a healthy diet, the calories need to be considered. You'll find 100 calories in your choice of 4oz wine, 12oz beer, or 1oz of liquor. Since alcohol is dehydrating, it's best to pair your drink with a glass of water.

- **Limit the salt.** Restaurants add more than enough salt to their cooking, so keep the salt shaker at a distance.

▶ **Select High Octane Fuel.** You wouldn't put sand and water into your gas tank and expect it to run, would you? Junk food isn't completely off-limits, but start with the healthy basics:

- **Up your intake of fruits and vegetables.** Fruits and vegetables provide a powerful dose of essential vitamins, minerals, and antioxidants and naturally aid in digestion since they're high in fiber. The National Cancer Institute (in association with other health groups) recommend at least five serving of fruits and vegetables a day to keep the doctor away, yet most of us average just half that. Fruits and vegetables protect us from cancer, lower high blood pressure, and keep our tummies trimmer. Travelers, even those who eat healthy at home, have a tendency to neglect the five-serving rule. To up your intake on the road, carry fresh and dried fruit with you, order a fresh fruit bowl for the hotel room, and request fresh fruit and veggies in restaurants even if it's not on the menu. If restaurants are offering cream of broccoli soup and fresh strawberries on the cheesecake, they'll probably serve you some steamed broccoli and a bowl of fresh strawberries if you ask.

- **Fill up on fiber.** Nutrition experts recommend we eat 20-35 gms of fiber each day, but most of us get less than half that amount. In addition to the five plus servings of fruits and vegetables, aim for three servings of whole grain breads and cereals. Add beans two times a week. If you find yourself feeling a bit more gassy, try a supplement called *Beano*® available in grocery stores.

Fiber Facts:

Fruits & vegetables	Each ½c serving of fresh or canned has 2 gms. Dried fruit has the same amount of fiber as the fresh version (15 raisins have the same amount of fiber as 15 grapes).
Whole grains	Most grain products offered (such as cereal, white rice, noodles, pizza crust, white bread and rolls) have only 0-1 gm fiber per serving. Whole grain breads have 2-3 gms/slice. Whole grain cereals have 3-9 gms (shredded wheat, raisin bran, oatmeal) per ½ cup serving.
Nuts	A small handful (¼c) has 2-3 gms of fiber. If you're watching your weight keep in mind it also contains 200-250 calories.

	Fiber Facts (cont.):
Popcorn	Each cup has a gram of fiber. Avoid the fat-ladened airport and movie theatre popcorn – a small box contains 440 calories and 30 gms of fat! Pack your own "light" microwave popcorn; many hotels have microwaves available.
Beans	They're not only high in fiber, they're a good source of protein too.

- **Eat protein-rich foods twice a day.** Protein is needed for healthy skin and muscles and to strengthen our immune systems. But unless you're a serious bodybuilder, you'll get plenty in just two 3oz servings a day (3oz is the size of a deck of cards). Good sources of protein include beef, pork, fish, shellfish, chicken, cheese, tofu, beans, and eggs. On a weekly basis, aim for at least two servings of fish and two servings of vegetarian protein (beans, egg whites, or tofu). Balance out the rest of the week with five servings of chicken or turkey and the remaining five servings from beef or pork.

- **Reinforce the body structure.** Milk and milk products are a great source of muscle-building protein and bone-strengthening calcium. Dairy products also appear to be helpful in lowering blood pressure. So drink two cups a day and go for the skim or lowfat variety to save fat and calories. Don't like milk? Refer to the section on "*Supplement with the Additives You Need*" for alternatives.

▶ **Limit the Less Nutritious Foods.**

- **Watch your sugar intake.** Sugar is considered "empty calories" since they contain calories but very little nutrients. To get enough of the healthy foods without eating too many calories, it's essential to keep your sugar intake to no more than 10% of total calories. For example, if you need 2000 calories to maintain your weight, sugar should be kept under 200 calories a day.

15

That's the amount of sugar in a medium sized soda, four cups of coffee with two heaping teaspoon of sugar in each, *or* an average size dessert. Unfortunately, sugar is not found in just the most obvious places, it's added to lots of foods such as bread, cereal, tomato sauce, coffee creamer, salad dressing, and coleslaw. If you're watching your sugar intake but crave something sweet, try eating a jawbreaker or hot ball. You'll get just two to three teaspoons of sugar in 30 minutes of tasty fun!

- **Trim the fat.** For reducing your risk of heart disease and cancer or to lose weight, health authorities suggest reducing the fat in your diet to no more than 30% of your total calories. Since the guideline is based on the total calories consumed, people who burn more calories can eat more fat.

Maximum Fat (gm) Intake:	
Inactive Women	50
Active Women	60-80
Inactive Men	60
Active Men	80-100

That may sound like a lot, but most of us eat more than that – especially when we eat out without making the changes discussed later in this chapter. Restaurants tend to serve large portions of meat, select fattier cuts, and add more fat than you would in your own kitchen. So in addition to limiting the animal protein to just 6oz a day, ask for it to be broiled, roasted, or grilled. Remove the skin from poultry and trim off all visible fat. Ask for lowfat or skim milk for drinking, in your cereal, or in your coffee, and limit the cheese since restaurants aren't using lowfat varieties. Lastly, ask for salad dressings, gravies, butters, and sauces to be served on the side so you can use less.

Fat Facts*:

Food	Fat (gm)
Fresh fruits and vegetables w/out added fats	0
6 oz of lean meat	20
6 oz fatty meat	50
1 scrambled *or* fried egg	8
1 teaspoon margarine, butter, oil	5
2 tablespoons sauce on meat, vegetables, etc	5-20
1 level tablespoon salad dressing	6-8
2 cups Fettuccine Alfredo	75
20 Mexican chips	20
Medium loaded baked potato	40
8 oz whole milk	8
Small box of popcorn	30
16 oz Latte	12
16 oz Mocha with whipped cream	20
Average fast food combo w/burger, fries	50
Average dessert	20-40
1 slice of cheese	10

*Excerpted from <u>Dining Lean–how to eat healthy in restaurants</u> by Dr. Joanne Lichten. In bookstores, online, or 888-431-5326.

▶ **Follow a Sensible Eating Plan**

• **Power up with protein, calm down with carbs.** If breakfast doesn't stick with you and leaves your stomach growling by mid-morning, try starting your day with an energizing breakfast containing a protein source such as eggs, egg substitutes, cottage cheese, *or* Canadian bacon. Then for lunch, eat your second serving of protein (such as lean chicken, beef, beans, tofu, *Gardenburgers*®). End the day with Mother Nature's sedative, a relaxing evening meal featuring plenty of cereal, rice, potatoes, noodles, and/or bread. Add veggies, but skip the meat.

• **Carbohydrates are not bad.** Surely you've seen the books that claim carbohydrates are fattening. They encourage a diet consisting of mostly meat and fat and tell you to stay away from the so-called "fattening" foods like sugar, starches, and fruits. Some of us are old enough to remember when this fad diet was popular (back in the 1970's) and then went out of favor. While you *can* lose weight on the program (or *any* other diet program that limits food choices for that matter), it's hard to stick to a restrictive program long-term. Besides, the low carbohydrate/high fat diet is unhealthy! With heart disease and cancer as our top two killers, it's essential to minimize our saturated fat intake and add plenty of nutritious fruits, vegetables, and whole grains.

- **Limit your calories if you're getting spare tires.** Remember that when we eat more calories than our bodies need, we deposit them as fat in our holding tanks. The only way to lose weight is to eat fewer calories or burn more calories than you currently do now. Research, as well as the 2000 National Nutrition Debate, has determined that it doesn't matter which nutrient you reduce (carbohydrates, proteins, or fat) as long as the total calories go down. However, additional research (including this author's) and data from the Weight Control Registry indicate that people who consume a high fiber, high carbohydrate, low fat diet tend to be leaner and more likely to maintain a significant weight loss.

- **Take Dr Jo's "No Big Deal" approach!** Whether you want to lose weight, lower your cholesterol, or get your diabetes under control – we know from research (and probably your own personal experience as well) that making major changes in your eating habits are difficult to maintain long term. People who have been successful at keeping excess weight off long-term continue to include their favorite foods since deprivation often leads to rebound bingeing and weight gain. Instead of vowing to give up all your favorites, give yourself permission to enjoy an occasional decadence while instituting a *few* small changes that are "no big deal" for you – those you can stick with long-term.

- **Eat your pleasers. Skip the teasers.** What are your pleasers – the foods you really love? Go ahead and enjoy them. Just don't waste your calories on the "teasers" – food that is conveniently there – like, perhaps, the airline peanuts or pretzels or candy at the hotel registration desk. Be picky about what you eat and you won't feel deprived!

- **Have fun and enjoy every bite!** Food is to be savored. Eat what you like, eat it slowly paying attention to when you've had enough, and don't feel guilty about eating the foods you love. There aren't any "forbidden" foods – it's the frequency and amount that really matters.

Dr Jo's "No Big Deal" Approach to Weight Loss:

1. Forget the latest fad diets. They don't work long-term and the rebounding weight gain is depressing.
2. Don't give up all your favorite foods or "pleasers." Instead have them just once or twice a week rather than every day.
3. Skip the "teasers" – those foods you eat just because they're there.
4. Institute a few small changes that are "no big deal" for you to make. These may include:
   Baked meats more often than fried
   A smaller portion of meat and more veggies
   Small fries rather than large
   Diet instead of regular soda (give your taste buds a couple of weeks to adjust)
   Black coffee instead of with cream and/or sugar
   Egg substitutes instead of eggs
   Fat-free or low-fat milk instead of regular
   Fat-free salad dressings instead of the regular
   Leaving one bite of everything on your plate!

Remember: cutting back just 100 calories a day will result in an almost effortless ten-pound weight loss in a year!

▶ **Supplement with the Additives You Need.** If all the car maintenance you ever do is add fuel, eventually your car will break down. Your car, like your body, needs other additives. Vitamins and minerals help us to utilize the energy from food and keep us healthy and strong. On the other hand, "to ignore diet and just use supplements is like putting on a seat belt and driving like a maniac," says vitamin researcher Paul Jacques of Tufts University.

- **Take a multivitamin and mineral supplement.** If you're always on the go, chances are you're not getting the recommended levels of the essential vitamins and minerals. There's no risk for normal healthy individuals to take a multivitamin and mineral pill containing no more than 100% of the daily requirements (such as *Centrum®*). Men and postmenopausal women should select one with less than 100% iron. For best absorption, take it with one of your larger meals.

- **But don't self-prescribe higher doses.** Medications carry a benefit at a prescribed dosage but can be dangerous when too much is taken. The same is true for vitamins and minerals – excessive supplementation can also impair our health. For example, over 100 mg vitamin B6 can lead to nonreversible nerve damage, over 2500 mg calcium or more than 2000 IU vitamin D can promote kidney stones, and high levels of folic acid (1000+ mg) can mask a dangerous vitamin B12 deficiency.

- **Take calcium supplements if you don't like milk.** Don't fall for the myth that adults don't need calcium, only kids. Bones are active cells just like the rest of the body and require calcium on a regular basis to replace its losses. Calcium not only prevents bone fractures, but is also important for blood coagulation, muscle contractions, and blood pressure control. Although dark, green leafy vegetables are high in calcium, most of us don't eat enough to make it count. It's recommended that we eat two (three for postmenopausal women) servings of milk products each day. One serving is 8oz milk,

8oz yogurt, or 1oz cheese. If you're not consuming enough, take a 500mg calcium supplement for each serving you missed. For best absorption, take just 500mg between each meal. The best absorbed calcium supplements are calcium citrate (such as *Citracal®*) or calcium carbonate (including chewable *Viactiv®* or *Tums®*). While vitamin D helps in the absorption of calcium, if your multivitamin/mineral pill contains vitamin D, get your calcium supplement without it.

- **Treat your lactose intolerance.** If you get stomach cramps and diarrhea when you consume milk products, your body may not be producing enough of the enzyme, lactase. Try taking *LactAid®* tablets with your meals containing milk or cheese. And drink *LactAid®* milk when you're at home.

- **Take a fiber supplement if needed.** If you don't get enough fiber or your doctor recommends a supplement, consider a product like *Metamucil®* which is also available in good-tasting (and easy to pack) wafers.

Defensive Dining

Road warriors eat out more often than homebodies – and that can negatively impact our health. Restaurants serve huge portions, add more fat, and offer only a limited number of healthy foods. But, eating away from home doesn't have to do you in. Whether you are feasting on a fabulous four course meal or fast food, here are some tips to get past that road block.

▶ **Get It Your Way.** You're paying for the meal and you have to wear the excess calories, so ask for it your way.

- **Special order it.** Don't settle for the usual preparation method if it doesn't fit into your plan. Ask for grilled chicken instead of fried on the salad, request less meat/ more veggies in your stirfry, and ask them to use broth instead of oil to sauté the vegetables.

- **Choose the lean, mean varieties.** When eating out, animal meats are the most readily available form of the protein. To reduce the artery-clogging cholesterol and

21

saturated fatty acids, order the leaner cuts, and request it baked, broiled, or roasted (rather than fried). Think of cheese as a condiment, not a meal. Although we can buy lowfat cheese in grocery stores, restaurants use the full-fat version (as high in fat as fried chicken). So consider the chicken enchiladas rather than cheese and ask for your pizza to be prepared "light" on the cheese.

- **Leave off the shine.** Have you ever noticed that restaurant food "shines?" That's all the added fat! Typically, steaks, fish, and chicken breasts are brushed with butter/oil before serving – say no to the added fat. Request your veggies to be served without the butter or cheese sauce and order your pancakes without the butter glob on top. Since upscale joints slather butter or oil on the your sandwich bun before it's grilled, be sure to tell them "I want my buns dry." Ask them to use a nonstick spray when they make your omelet (they use it to make the waffles, so they'll have the spray).

- **Get it on the side.** Every tablespoon of mayonnaise, salad dressing, butter, & oil contains about 100 calories. Don't let the guy in the back of the kitchen decide your pants or dress size. Ask for salad dressings and fish toppings, potato and veggie toppings "on the side." Use the dip and stab method to enjoy the taste without putting your fat cells on alert. Dip your fork into the dressing, then into the salad for a taste with every bite.

- **Make Miss Manners mad.** You have *my* permission to play with your food. Trim off the visible fat on the meat, pull off the chicken skin, scrape off the breading or excess sauce, and drain off the excess butter or oil. Perhaps "Miss Manners" would object, but she doesn't have to fit into your jeans.

▶ **Control Your Portions.** Sometimes it's hard to resist food that is sitting right in front of you – especially when Mom taught you to clean your plate. But Mom will forgive you if you make the healthy choice to eat only as much as you're genuinely hungry for since eating more won't help the starving children of the world. Here's how to do it without a guilt trip.

- **Tell them how much you want.** Order ala carte if possible so you get just what you want. Or if the Mexican platter comes with three enchiladas, ask for just two. You might still have to pay the full price, but you've saved yourself from overeating.

- **Split it with a friend.** If you're traveling with a friend or family member, consider sharing a plate with them and ordering an extra portion of veggies. Since most restaurant-sized desserts are 300 to over 1000 calories each, share them as well.

- **Hold the bread.** Do you start your meals at home with slices of bread and butter or chips and dips? Probably not. This habit alone could add on several hundred calories. If you're dining alone, consider calling your order in ahead of time so it's ready when you are seated (and there's no time for the chips).

- **Get dessert on the road.** The great thing about enjoying an occasional dessert in a restaurant (rather than at home) – is that the rest of the pie or cake isn't sitting there "haunting" you.

- **Get the doggie bag *with* dinner.** This is the ultimate portion control device. Put away part of your meal right when it arrives on your table. Close the box and set it aside. Out of sight, out of mind really does work! If your hotel room doesn't have a refrigerator, just leave the box behind or give it to the next homeless person you see.

- **Have closure to the meal.** Most of us need a signal that the meal is over. For many of us, it is when the food is gone and the plate is empty. But since restaurants tend to serve us more than we need to eat, using

23

that signal is a prescription for weight gain. Instead, ask the server to take the plate away when you are comfortably full. If the server is no where in sight, place your napkin on top of the plate or set it on an empty table nearby. Or eliminate the temptation to keep nibbling by making your food unpalatable by salting it heavily or pouring on the hot sauce. I order hot tea as my closing signal; others like to have a mint.

▶ **Check the Price Tag.** When you go shopping for a car, do you ever look at the price tag? Sure you do. Chances are you examine the features and then ask yourself if it's worth the price. If you need to watch your weight, it's time to look at food in the same way. You don't have to be a walking calorie-counter, but when you find out a large cinnamon roll has over 800 calories and more than a half a stick of butter, it may make you think twice (or at least it may encourage you to split it with a friend).

- **Pick Up *Dining Lean*.** My other book, *Dining Lean: how to eat healthy in your favorite restaurant*, is a 304 page book that offers a much expanded version of this chapter. There you'll discover that an oat bran muffin can be more fattening than a chocolate éclair and that frying will double or triple the calories of any food. *Dining Lean*'s detailed nutritional information of more than a thousand menu items reveals that one "loaded" nacho has more than 100 calories and your morning mocha contains more than 300 calories. Look up your favorite foods and then ask yourself if it's worth it.
- **Get the facts**. Removing the skin from poultry will cut the fat content in half. But since skinless chicken tends to absorb more fat when deep-fried, it's no healthier than the regular fried chicken. Salads aren't always healthy either. The taco salad, at one fast food Mexican restaurant, is the highest calorie item on the menu! Even a green salad doused with 250 calories worth of fat-laden dressing isn't a wise choice considering what little fiber and other nutrients that you'll find in the iceberg

lettuce. While bagels can be healthy, they're just bread – and lots of it. The standard deli-sized bagel is the equivalence of four to five slices of bread. Also, since we hear much about olive oil being healthy, keep in mind that at 120 calories per tablespoon, it's just as fattening as the other oils.

- **Eat out and lose weight.** You know that it's possible to eat healthy in restaurants, but did you know that you can lose weight too? *Dr. Jo's Eat Out & Lose Weight Plan* (at the end of this chapter) tells you exactly which choices will keep your motor running and eliminate those spare tires.

▶ **Boost Your Breakfast**

- **Go with fresh fruit instead of juice.** Although both are high in vitamins and minerals, juice is void of any substantial amount of fiber. For those concerned with their weight, juice has the same number of calories as soda (about 150 calories/12oz). A fresh orange has just 60 – and it can be more satisfying since it takes longer to eat.

- **Try egg substitutes.** Egg substitutes are just as high in protein as eggs yet weigh in at just a third of the calories (because most brands leave out the egg yolk). Greatly improved over the years, it's difficult to taste the difference when you add the veggies and perhaps a small amount of cheese. No egg substitutes available? Ask for scrambled egg whites. And don't forget to ask them to use a nonstick spray.

- **Bacon is better than sausage.** While Canadian bacon or ham is often a lean cut, all the other breakfast meats are very high in fat. If you must have one of the other meats, consider that two slices of thin bacon has just 70 calories and 6 gms of fat while sausage contains 200 calories and 16 gms fat in the usual two patty serving.

- **Choose whole grain bread.** Have you ever wondered why biscuits and croissants are so flaky? It's the mul-

25

tiple layers of fat separating the flour. Sometimes they don't look greasy but it's just the dry-feeling hydrogenated shortening that's fooling you. Biscuits and croissants have at least 50% more calories than toast or English muffins. Instead, order whole wheat toast and remember to order it dry so you can control the toppings.

- **Avoid dessert at breakfast.** If you've been getting the mid-morning slumps, opt for something healthier than a high sugar/high fat pastry for breakfast. Or if you must, keep it small. The fluffy yeast doughnuts have 200 calories each, cake doughnuts have 300, and a medium danish has a belt-stretching 400 calories.

- **Pick a healthy cereal.** As mentioned earlier, shredded wheat, raisin bran, and oatmeal are the highest fiber cereals commonly available in restaurants. *Wheaties®* and *Cheerios®*, though not as high in fiber, are good choices since they're made with whole grain and are low in sugar. The other plain or sugared cereals can qualify as a low calorie breakfast since they contain just 100 calories per cup, but because they're nearly void of fiber they may cause your stomach to start growling mid-morning. Adding dried fruit and nuts, while healthy, can jump the calories up – granola contains 250 calories in just a ½ cup serving! Don't forget to request skim milk.

- **Watch the butter and syrup**. Three (4") pancakes have just 330 calories and a (7") round Belgian waffles contains 500 calories. Not too bad, but adding butter and syrup more than doubles the calories. At about 200 calories each, take your pick: butter, syrup, or whipping cream – not all three! If you want to cut back on the syrup calories, here are your options. You can do the "dip and stab" with your pancake syrup or ask for sugar-free syrup (most restaurants have it). I like to mix the regular syrup with the sugar-free – then it's close to the "Lite" syrup available at grocery stores.

- **Get it plain.** While coffee and tea are nearly calorie-free, the addition of sugar, cream, flavorings, and whipping cream can cause spare tires where you never had them. Years ago I had a patient visit me complaining that she had gained 10 pounds over the past year. Although she assured me that nothing had changed in her diet or exercise routine (she figured it was her metabolism), the cause soon became evident. She had begun a traveling job early that year. Back in her home office, she would use four tablespoons of skim milk (throughout the day) in her coffee. But, on the road, she would use what ever was available – usually cream, whole milk, or one of those flavored creamers. That small change added up to an extra 100 calories a day or 36,500 calories over a year! Once she realized what a big difference a little thing can make, she chose to drink her coffee black and lost the ten pounds. It usually takes just a couple of weeks to get used to the taste difference. P.S. Think twice before you squirt on the whipping cream; that ½ cup squirt adds another 100 calories and 7 gms of saturated fat!

▶ **Order a Lean Lunch**
- **Enjoy the ultimate lean lunch.** A small grilled or roasted chicken sandwich (without mayo or sauce) has about 300 calories, while the larger ones have about 400. Remember that upscale restaurants are buttering the bun – ask for it dry to save 100 calories. By the way, if the chicken sandwich (or fish for that matter) is described as "crispy", it's not grilled. Those fried chicken or fish sandwiches have an extra 100-200 calories – with nearly all the extra calories coming from fat!
- **Get a small, plain burger.** A burger once or twice a week offers you variety and an extra boost of iron over the chicken. The "kid-sized" plain (mustard, ketchup, and pickles) burgers contain approximately 300 calories and the quarter pounders weigh in at about 450 calories. Avoid the "big" burgers – they range anywhere from 650 calories for the one third pound to nearly 1000 calories for the half pound burgers. For flavor with few

27

calories, try adding BBQ sauce or salsa.

- **Deli-sliced meats can be lean.** In fact, a small bun, pita, or six inch sub filled with chicken, turkey, ham, seafood, or roast beef and without dressing, mayo, or oil will only have about 300-400 calories. The larger buns and foot-long subs can healthily fill a bigger appetite at 600-800 calories.

- **Mayonnaise or french fries – take your pick.** As you can see, a sandwich consisting of lean meat and bread is often very lean. It's the extras that add on the calories and the fat. Since most of us can't afford to eat as many calories as we might want, it's important to rank our priorities. For approximately 100 calories each, you can have: a tablespoon of mayonnaise or salad dressing, a slice of cheese, a couple strips of bacon, sauteed mushrooms, sliced avocado or guacamole, a single large onion ring, seven potato puffs, 10 regular fries, or 20 skinny french fries. How many of these can you (calorically) afford?

- **Go for the salad.** Lettuce and raw veggies are nearly calorie-free. Add a bit of sliced chicken and some fat-free or lowfat dressing and you have a healthy lunch. To round out a healthy salad meal, add a few crackers (about 10-15 calories each) or a roll (200 calories) for some carbohydrates. But not all salads are healthy. If you allow the restaurant to put the dressing on your salad, chances are they will put three tablespoons on a small salad and up to a half cup (over 500 calories of grease!) on a large salad.

- **Examine your fluids.** All sodas are fat-free but only diet sodas are calorie-free. A large fountain beverage at your favorite fast food restaurant has about 300 calories. A police officer once told me that his weight had gotten so high that he was told that he'd have to be moved to a desk job if he didn't take off some weight. For his "no big deal" approach, he switched to diet sodas, and over the next year, lost 87 pounds!

▶ **Delicious Dinner Options**

- **Pass the bread basket.** Or take just a slice or two and hand the basket back to the server. Since butters and oils (even the healthier ones) contain 100 calories per level tablespoon, it's best to enjoy just a thin smear or dip rather than a soaking.

- **Broth-based soups are the healthiest.** At fewer than 150 calories a cup, they're lower in fat and calories than the cream-based soups (at 200-400 calories/cup). The French Onion Soup may be broth-based but it's prepared with so much butter that it weighs in at close to 400 calories per cup. If you opt for the high fat soup, order the cup instead of the bowl and if the tomato soup is pink rather than red, it's a sure bet that it's been prepared with milk or cream (the more you've paid for the soup, the more likely it's cream).

- **Skip the appetizer or make it your entrée.** Did you know that each single buffalo wing, stuffed jalapeno, or fried mozzarella stick with sauce has about 100 calories? If you want more than one or two, you may want to consider the high fat/high calorie appetizers as your entrée. These healthier appetizers also make great entrees: shrimp cocktail, Thai summer rolls, chicken satays (Asian-style grilled chicken on skewers), sushi, steamed vegetable dumplings, and the margarita pizza ("light on the cheese, please").

- **Choose the leanest protein for dinner.** We all know that white chicken and fish (prepared without added fat) are lean. But did you know that lean cuts of beef (sirloin steak, filet, London broil, New York, Club, kabob, Delmonico) and pork (tenderloin) are also acceptable on a healthy diet? Remember to keep your combined protein portion to 6 oz *a day* and ask for the grilled, steamed, or roasted versions.

- **Request the sauces, butters, toppings "on the side."** Save 100 calories or more by asking for your meat, potato, and vegetables without all the butter and sauces (or get it on the side if you're worried about the meat being too dry). Vegetable and fruit salsas are wonderful, lowfat flavor enhancers.

- **Demand more veggies.** Restaurants often serve large portions of meat, smaller portions of starches, and very little if any vegetables. Nutritionally, those proportions are all wrong – much like an inverted food pyramid. You'll be doing your heart and intestinal tract (not to mention your belly roll) a favor by asking for half the meat and double the vegetables. Even if vegetables are not on the menu, they're nearly always available for the asking.

▶ Choose Healthy Chinese

- **Skip the buffet.** Remember what we said about shiny food? Have you looked at the buffet? The extra oil may be helpful to prevent the food from sticking to the pan but it makes *you* start sticking in those tiny airline seats. Being in a hurry can make the buffet all the more tempting. Why not call your order from the hotel or meeting room, then drive over (or better yet, walk) to the restaurant? It'll be ready when you arrive.

- **Eat *authentic* Chinese food.** The real stuff consists of a little bit of meat, chicken, or other protein source stir-fried with lots of veggies in a small amount of oil. But that's typically not the way it's prepared at your favorite "Americanized-Chinese" restaurant. Dishes often contain more meat than vegetables and instead of a couple of teaspoons of oil, some restaurants use as much as a quarter of a cup (500 calories worth)! Since each meal is made to order, request more veggies and less meat in your favorite dish and ask them to use as little oil as possible.

- **Order steamed white rice rather than fried rice.** Even if the plate is typically served with fried rice, ask for the steamed rice. Fried rice has 50% more calories – all coming from fat!

- **Stay away from the deep fried meats.** We all know that beef has more fat and calories than white chicken. But what makes a bigger impact is whether it is stir-fried or deep fat fried. So stay away from deep-fried entrees like Sweet 'n Sour or Lemon Chicken (look for the words "crispy" or "fried" in the description). These dishes are nearly 100% meat (0% vegetables) and they're fried, resulting in three to four times more calories than a mixed, non-fried order. I also found out that many Chinese restaurants, in order to get the food out faster, will deep fry all the meats (not enough that it's crispy). Avoid restaurants that serve the food up too fast.

- **Watch the extras.** Just a sprinkling of nuts (¼ cup) or a half cup of crunchy chow mein noodles can add on another 200-250 calories. Ask for Jicama or waterchestnuts for crunch instead. Go ahead and enjoy the fortune cookie; it's just about fat-free and only 30 calories.
- **Use chopsticks.** If you're inexperienced with using chopsticks you will find it difficult to eat quickly. This allows time for your stomach to signal when you're full.

▶ **Japanese Restaurants**
- **Share your dish.** For four people, order three dishes including a vegetable meal. And since most dishes are heavy on the meat, don't be shy to ask for more veggies in the stir fried dishes.
- **Stay away from fried foods.** Each piece of tempura (fried vegetable pieces) contains about 50 calories and 3 gms fat.
- **Go for the low fat foods.** Order Yakitori (meat on a skewer), steamed rice, and stir-fried vegetables for a healthy, low calorie meal. Sushi is another lean option. Not all sushi is raw; sushi bars also offer: scrambled eggs, smoked or broiled eel, smoked salmon, boiled shrimp, crab, and fried tofu. Each piece has just 30-50 calories. The dipping sauce made of ginger, horseradish, and soy sauce is negligible in calories, but high in sodium (you might want to ask for the low sodium soy sauce). Other healthy options are nonfried vegetable

31

spring or summer rolls, steamed dumplings, or miso hot pot (vegetables with noodles). Try the soba (wheat) noodles instead of the udon (white noodles). The tomato miso soup, looks creamy, but it's not fattening. Other low cal soups include Won Ton or Udon Noodle soup – at just 200-300 calories in a large bowl! Like Chinese restaurants, Japanese restaurants (especially the Japanese steakhouses that cook at your table) add much more oil for stir frying than required.

▶ **Lean Mean, Mexican Cuisine**

- **Count your chips.** Each large restaurant-style chip has 25 calories and one gm fat. Eat the whole basket and you've consumed as much fat as a half of a stick of butter! Some upscale Mexican restaurants offer baked chips which contain about half the calories and negligible fat. But don't expect it to be on the menu, you'll have to ask. Another flavorful option is to dip corn tortillas into the salsa instead of chips.

- **Go heavy on the salsa.** Enjoy it mild or wild! Either way, salsa is very low in calories and high in vitamin C and antioxidants. Guacamole, on the other hand, contains nearly 30 calories per level tablespoon! Oh, and that creamy green sauce? That contains guacamole too.

- **Order ala carte.** A typical Mexican platter has 1000-1500 calories or more. So order ala carte to get only what you really love! Do you like fajitas but tend to nibble at the beans and rice just because they're there? Next time, order just the tacos al carbon (fajita meat in a flour tortilla).

- **Ask for the bean soup.** Most Mexican restaurants offer refried beans with meals. They're loaded with fat (20 gms) – and most often it's lard (a heart-risky saturated fat). Instead, ask for black beans, beans ala charro, or bean soup. Because these offerings are lower in fat, you'll cut the calories in half. When eating the bean soup, skim off the beans and leave the bacon-rich broth in the cup.

- **A single tortilla is not fattening, but how many can you eat**? A small corn tortilla is just about fat-free and has 50 calories while the small flour tortilla has about 100 calories and 3 gms fat. Frying the tortillas can double the calories – while one of those puny fried taco shells contains 50, a large fried taco salad shell contains over 400 calories. Depending on your calorie needs and the balance of your meal, two or three flour tortillas are probably enough.

- **Not too much cheese.** Cheese is an excellent protein source; ounce for ounce it has as much protein as fish, chicken, and beef. But the cheese offered in restaurants contains 10 gms of fat in every ounce (one slice or two tablespoons shredded). Protein sources ranked from leanest to those highest in fat include: grilled fish, chicken breast or fajitas, beef fajitas, ground beef, and then cheese. So choose the chicken enchiladas rather than cheese and chicken fajita salad instead of the ground beef taco salad. With each healthier choice you'll save about half the calories (all from the fat reduction).

- **Beware of the sizzle.** Ever wonder why the fajitas "sizzle" on the way to the table? You guessed it! It's all the butter or oil used. And if you thought the chicken fajitas were leaner, take a look. While the beef fajitas produce enough shine on their own (or with a light brushing), restaurants often pour butter on the chicken to prevent it from looking so dry. Ask them not to "pretty up" your dishes with all that extra oil.

- **Little things can really add up.** While two beef fajitas tacos with lettuce, tomato, onion contain just 400 calories (and 19 gms of fat), adding just a level tablespoon of guacamole, sour cream, and shredded cheese to each taco will double the fat and add on an extra 200 calories! So limit yourself to just the toppings you really love.

How to Stay Healthy & Fit on the Road

▶ **Italian Restaurants**

- **Fill up on bean soup and salad.** Don't let the healthy sounding "vinaigrette" name confuse you. It's the same as Italian dressing at 75 calories a tablespoon! Even a small salad has three tablespoons; larger salads have more. You always order it "on the side," don't you?

- **Request pasta with tomato sauce.** The average dinner serving of two cups of pasta with tomato or marinara sauce contains just 580 calories. But you'll get 700 calories with clam sauce, 950 with meat sauce, 1000 with pesto sauce, and over 1200 calories with Alfredo or Carbonara sauce. Don't be shy about asking for a different sauce. For example, request your primavera to be prepared with a tomato sauce rather than the cream sauce.

- **Lighten up the creamy stuff.** If you really must have one of the creamy sauces, ask them to put on just half the usual amount. Ask for some extra sauce on the side if you're concerned that it may be too dry. Chances are you'll find a lighter, still flavorful (and now healthier) pasta.

- **Select a nonfried entree.** Veal, chicken, or eggplant parmigiana is breaded, fried, and then covered with tomato sauce and cheese. Some Italian restaurants may be willing to grill it instead of frying, ask. If not, stick with a lower fat pasta dish or grilled fish.

- **Order a luncheon or appetizer portion.** Many Italian restaurants can accomodate – even if it's not mentioned on the menu. So if you're really in the mood for eggplant parmigiana, get the *appetizer* portion.

- **Get less meat.** At dinner, meat portions are large – more protein than you need for the whole day. If you want meat, consider ordering a pasta dish that contains some meat rather than a meat entree.

- **Cut the oil.** Upscale restaurants use a lot of oil to cook the accompanying veggies & meat before adding the sauce and the noodle. Since they are preparing the dish fresh for you, ask them to cook the veggies and meat in broth or wine for a 200 calorie savings (and still great taste). Don't forget to ask for your side dish of vegetables to be steamed without butter or oil. Otherwise, plan on another 100+ calories.

▶ Dr Jo's Pizza Prescription

- **Choose a healthy, low fat pizza crust.** How do you know? If your pizza leaves a ring on the cardboard box and shiny fingers, it's not low fat. Some crusts are made with so much fat that they might as well be fried! These high fat crusts have as much as 30% more calories, so find a brand that passes the ring test.

- **Stick with the regular or thin crusts.** They're much lower in fat and calories than the deep dish or stuffed pizza crusts.

- **Ask for tomato sauce.** Some of the more upscale Italian restaurants may use oil or a cream sauce.

- **Order it with low fat toppings.** Instead of sausage and pepperoni, try some of the no fat toppings such as peppers, onions, mushrooms, pineapple, spinach, and tomato slices. Moderate fat toppings consist of Canadian bacon, ham, grilled chicken, and olives.

- **Go "light" on the cheese.** Order your pizza "light on the cheese" and you'll cut another 40-50 calories on each slice. OK, at least don't ask for "extra cheese."

- **Put all these suggestions together.** Two slices of a large Supreme pizza have 900 calories and 39 gms fat. When you order the same size pizza with no-fat veggies and request the pizza to be made "light on the cheese," these two slices now have just 500 calories and 10 gms fat.

▶ Airline Food

- **Limit yourself to one snack.** Oh sure, nuts contain healthy monounsaturated fats and pretzels are low in fat. But combine dehydrated travelers with the low humidity on the plane – and the last thing we need is more salt! If you want it anyway, consider that each tiny little bag of nuts or pretzels contains about 100 calories.

- **Special order your meal.** When making your airline reservation, check to see if a meal is being served. If there is, be sure to order a special meal. Not only are they healthier, they usually taste better. There are many choices – consider ordering low fat/low cholesterol, low calories, diabetic, high fiber, skinless/boneless chicken, vegetarian, Asian vegetable, Hindu, Moslem, Japanese, seafood (often cold shrimp), kosher, or the fruit plate. Most need only a 24 hour notice.

- **Redefine what you need for a meal.** Restaurants have spoiled us with huge portions so people often complain about the tiny flight meals, but it's really quite adequate for our needs. A recent economy meal contained 2 crackers, a small cube of cheese, a tiny granola bar, a mini box of raisins, and a bite size candy bar. That's about 350 calories – about what we burn in 4 hours of sitting.

Meals on Wheels

While it's possible to eat healthy in restaurants, sometimes it's just easier to bring some foods along for when flights are delayed, you need a quick snack, or if you just don't want to stop to eat. If you don't have any more room in your suitcase, considering going grocery shopping along the way or at your destination.

▶ **Pack Your Eating Essentials.** So you're ready for any situation, bring along:

- **Heating coil and insulated plastic cup** for heating water.
- **Large 16 oz plastic cup.** The products sold in convenient, paper cups that require just the addition of hot water are bulky to pack (and are a mess when they spill). Instead, pour the contents into a baggie and use your large plastic cup for preparation.
- **Small plastic plate**
- **Eating utensils**

▶ **Reach for these Healthy, Packable Foods** when you're stomach starts growling (no refrigeration needed):

- **Charlie's Light Lunch** (kit containing canned tuna or chicken, crackers, light mayonnaise, relish, and spoon).
- **Dehydrated, healthy soups.** Select from several high protein, high fiber soups including as *Nile Spice®*, *Fantastic®*, or *Healthy Choice®*. Just add hot water.
- **"Dr Jo's Breakfast in a Cup."** Pack in a baggie, 1/3c of both quick cooking oatmeal and nonfat dry milk powder, a mini box of raisins, and a teaspoon of sugar (package of sweetener). Add a cup of boiling water for a filling, nutritious, and quick breakfast.
- **Instant hot cereals** such as oatmeal, grits, or cream of wheat. The most nutritious is oatmeal since it's a good source of fiber. *Health Valley®* and *Nabsico®* Harvest Morning packs flavored oatmeal in a paper cup.
- **Instant mashed potatoes**. Also available in disposable paper cups.
- **Fresh or dried fruit** (P.S. there are more choices than just raisins).
- **Dry cereals** like *Quaker®* Oat Bran or frosted mini shredded wheat.
- **Light microwave popcorn.** If there isn't a microwave oven in your room, check the vending room, or in the breakfast nook of the lobby.
- **Canned kippers, sardines, or oysters on crackers**
- **Bagels.**
- **Cookies** such as animal crackers, *Teddy Grahams®*
- **Crackers** including gold fish and *Triscuit®*.
- **Unsalted nuts** in a healthy trail mix.
- **Coffee or tea**. Pack your own to save money and time or take herbal and decaffeinated tea bags which are often not available.
- **Instant beverages** such as sugar-free *Crystal Light®*, *Koolaid®*, or hot cocoa.
- **Meal replacement bars and snack bars.** For a 100-150 calorie snack, opt for: *Health Valley®* Granola Bar (nearly all carbs with 3 gms of fiber), *Tiger's Milk* (55%

carbs), *Ensure®* (higher in protein), or *Glucerna®* (for people with diabetes) bar. If you need a 180-250 calorie meal replacement bar, try: *Balance® Bars* (promoting a 40/30/30 ratio of carbs, protein, &fats), *Powerbars®* (75% carbs, 3 gms fiber), *Clif® Bar* (65% carbs, 18% protein), *SlimFast®* (lower protein), or *Boost®* bars (61% carbs, 8% protein, and 33% fat). *Jenny Craig®* bars and *Clif®'s Luna Bars* also contain a well-balanced ratio of 58% carbs, 22% protein, and 20% fat. My favorites are *Clif®'s* Carrot Cake and *Balance®* Yogurt Honey Peanut.

Meal Replacement Bars: Do They Live Up to Their Name?

Meal replacement bars usually start with a healthy protein base consisting of soy protein, whey protein isolate, and skim milk powder. Some of the carbohydrates come from healthy peanuts, oatmeal, soy flour, and dried fruit. But most are in the form of non-nutritive sugars including brown rice syrup, evaporated can juice, corn syrup, and fructose. Though the bars are fairly low in fat (3-6 gms), it's surprising that often half of that amount is from unhealthier saturated fats such as palm kernel oil, chocolate, and cocoa butter.

From the nutritional information you'll see that this isn't really a "meal." You'll get the same nutritional value from grabbing a half pint of skim or reduced fat milk, a multi-vitamin/mineral supplement; and one of the following: a *Kudo®* bar, one long Fig Newton bar, an original size Rice Krispy Treat, or one thin *Nature Valley®* Granola Bar. P.S. the Fig Newtons and *Nature Valley®* bars are packed two to a package.

Not really healthy, right? But I still keep a meal replacement bar in my briefcase for emergencies. They take up little room, don't crush easily, need no refrigeration, and they hit the spot when I need some calories. But don't confuse them with a real meal!

▶ **Go Grocery Shopping or Pack a Cooler.** Before you embark on a road trip, freeze the bottles of water or juice (add ice as needed). If you're flying, shop for your own favorite foods when you arrive. If you don't have a car, ask the concierge if there is a market nearby that you can walk or take a taxi to. Hotels often supply small refrigerators for a small charge or for free; request them when you're making the reservation. Or when you're at the grocery store, buy an inexpensive styrofoam cooler that you can leave behind. Are you on a eating program that requires special foods? Reserve a room with a refrigerator and microwave, then have the food shipped directly to your hotel. Here are some ideas of healthy foods that require refrigeration:

- **Fresh fruit**
- **Diet sodas**
- **Skim milk** – for drinking or cereal
- **Fruit juices** – select those that contain 100% juice
- **Lowfat cheese**. There are some lowfat cheeses available in sticks or single portion balls.
- **Yogurt in a cup.** If you're watching your weight, choose the lowfat, low sugar varieties
- **Raw vegetables** such as mini carrots, broccoli, and snap peas
- **Salad in a bag** with light salad dressing
- **Luncheon deli meats** such as turkey, ham, lean roast beef or turkey pastrami.
- **Cottage cheese and fruit combos** in a cup
- **Cooked shrimp and red cocktail sauce**
- **Deli salads** such as coleslaw and bean salad – drained well
- **Roasted chicken.** Remove skin and fat before eating.

Dr Jo's Eat Out & Lose Weight Plan

I so often hear people say "I can't lose weight – I eat out often." But that isn't true! You can lose weight if you simply select meals that contain fewer calories than your daily maintenance calorie needs. To make it easy for you, I've developed some meal plans and these simple guidelines:

▶ **Make Only Slight Changes.** People who lose weight slowly are more are successful at keeping off the weight. Don't even try to lose more than a pound or two a week. Remember, don't give up all your favorite foods. And read the next chapter about how to burn more calories too.

▶ **Use the Chart Below for a Suggested Plan.** Begin by selecting meals from the suggested "fuel" sources. All of the "Regular Fuel" menu ideas contain 300-400 calories, "Super Fuel" contains 500-600 calories, and the "Premium Fuel" meals have 700-800 calories in each meal. Foods on the snack list weigh in at 100 calories each.

	Regular	Super	Premium	Snacks
Inactive Women	3	-	-	1
Active Women	1	2	-	3
Inactive Men	1	2	-	3
Active Men	-	1	2	3

▶**Keep Fat to 30% of Total.** As mentioned earlier, health authorities recommend getting no more than 30% of our daily calories from fat. Though the recommendation doesn't apply to each and every meal (just the average), for simplicity most of the meals were planned to contain no more than 30%. Those meals that are higher in fat are signified with an asterisk (*). Try to select no more than 1 higher fat meal per day.

▶ **Drink Plenty of Fluids.** Water, black coffee and tea, sugar sweeteners, and other diet beverages are calorie-free and may be consumed as desired.

▶**Feel Free to Make Substitutions.** Obviously, some of these items are more nutritious, but any of these can be substituted for another at approximately 100 calories each:

8oz fat-free or 1% milk
¾c or piece of fresh fruit
2t margarine or butter
2T cream cheese, pancake syrup, jelly or jam
8oz juice or regular soda
8oz mocha latte made w/skim milk
16oz cappuccino made w/skim milk
4oz wine, 8oz beer, or 1oz liquor
1T mayo
1 slice cheese, 2 strips bacon
10 french fries or 20 skinny fries

▶ **Choose from Snacks (100-150 calories) Including:**

Fruit, large piece
100% Fruit Juice, 8 oz
Light Popcorn, ½ bag
Health Valley® **granola bar or a snack bar such as** *Tiger's Milk*®, *Ensure*®, **or** *Glucerna*®.
½ *Clif*®, *Powerbar*®, *Luna*®, *Jenny Craig*®, *Balance*® **or other approximately 200 calorie bar.**
Raisins, small box
Bagel, ½ medium or 1/3 large
Light yogurt, 8oz container
Milk, 8oz carton of skim or lowfat
Frozen yogurt, 4oz kid's size
Pretzels or Peanuts, airline sized bag
Sugar-free hot cocoa, cup
Hot Cereal, instant oatmeal, cream of wheat, or grits packet

c=cup, lg=large, med= medium, oz=ounce, sl=slice, sm=small,
SW=sandwich, t=teaspoon, T=tablespoon, w/=with, w/out = without

How to Stay Healthy & Fit on the Road

▶ **Breakfast Ideas:**

Regular Breakfast Fuel (300-400 calories):

Fast food. 8oz 1% milk, 8oz juice, *or* piece of fresh fruit & one of the following fast food breakfast sandwiches: *Au Bon Pain*® Spinach & Cheese Croissant, *Del Taco*® Breakfast Burrito, *Jack in the Box*® Breakfast Jack, *Krystal*® Sunriser, *McDonald's* Egg McMuffin®, *Taco Bell*® Country Breakfast Burrito *or* Fiesta Breakfast Burrito, *WhatABurger*® Egg Omelet

Pancakes. Two 4 inch pancakes ("no butter on top"), 2T syrup, ½c melon

Yeast raised doughnut, 8oz juice *or* fresh fruit

Eggbeaters®, 2 prepared w/ "non-stick spray" please, 1sl Canadian bacon, 1sl lightly buttered wheat toast

Cereal: 1½c raisin bran or shredded wheat, ¾c lowfat milk, banana

English muffin w/2t jelly *or* jam, 1 scrambled egg, sm juice

Bagel. 1 sm (½ lg) w/1T cream cheese, piece of fresh fruit

Oatmeal. 1c w/½c skim milk, 2T raisins, 2T brown sugar

*****Biscuit, plain croissant *or* cake doughnut** (med.)

Super Breakfast Fuel (500-600 calories):

Fast food. One fast food breakfast SW listed under Regular Fuel *plus* 1c 1% milk *and* piece of fresh fruit

Vegetable *Eggbeater*® omelet (w/ "non-stick" spray) with cheese, side order tomatoes, 2 "dry" toast *or* English muffin with jam, 1c mixed fruit

Belgian waffle ("no butter on top"), ¼ syrup *or* 1c applesauce

1½c Raisin bran or shredded wheat, ¾ c lowfat milk, fresh fruit, 2 sl lightly buttered toast

Large deli bagel, lightly buttered or with thin smear cream cheese, piece of fresh fruit

Pancakes, three 4" ("no butter"), 3T syrup, ½c melon

*****2 eggs**, "dry" toast, 2 slices bacon, ½c juice

*****Higher fat fast food.** Pick one: Bacon/egg/cheese biscuit, croissant breakfast SW *or* sausage/egg biscuit

---

c=cup, lg=large, med= medium, oz=ounce, sl=slice, sm=small,
SW=sandwich, t=teaspoon, T=tablespoon, w/=with, w/out = without

Premium Breakfast Fuel (700-800 calories):

Double any of the **Regular Fuel** menu choices, including 2 of the Fast Food breakfast sandwiches

Bagel. 1 large deli-sized, 2T cream cheese, 8oz fat-free milk, piece of fresh fruit

2 scr or fried eggs, three 4" pancakes ("no butter on top"), ¼c syrup, 1c fruit

Vegetable *Eggbeater*® omelet ("use non-stick" spray) w/out cheese, sliced tomatoes, hashbrowns, 2 "dry" toast *or* English muffin w/jam, 1c mixed fruit

Medium-sized danish, muffin, cinnamon roll, *or* **croissant** plus 20oz latte made w/skim milk and piece of fresh fruit

▶ **Lunch Options:**

Regular Lunch Fuel (300-400 calories):

Sm grilled chicken sandwich (such as *Arby's*® light, *Carl Jr's*® BBQ, *KFC*® Tender Roast or Honey BBQ, *McDonald's*®, or *Wendy's*®) with little or no sauce

Small grilled chicken salad with fat-free dressing such as *Applebee's*® Lowfat Blackened, *Arby's*® Light Grilled, *Bob's Big Boy*® Chicken Breast, *Carl Jr's*® BBQ Chargrilled Chicken, *or Chick-fil-A*® Chick-n-Strips® Salad Plate.

6" Sub w/mustard or low-fat mayonnnaise or oil such as *Subway*® Veggie Delite, Turkey Breast, Ham, Roast Beef, *Subway Club*®, *Tuna or *Seafood & Crab® made with light mayo

Small *Gardenburger*® on bun with mustard, lettuce, tomato, onion.

Pizza. 2 lg slices of thin crust onion/mushroom/pepper/ham pizza "light on the cheese"

Sushi. 10 pieces with soy sauce, horseradish, and ginger

Chicken Fajita Pita (*Jack in the Box*® or *WhatABurger*®)

Fazoli's® **spaghetti** with tomato sauce or meat sauce

Applebee's® **Lowfat Veggie Quesadilla**

Au Bon Pain® **Oriental Chicken Salad** *or* *Mozzarella & Roasted Pepper Salad w/Fat Free Tomato Basil dressing

c=cup, lg=large, med≈ medium, oz=ounce, sl=slice, sm=small, SW=sandwich, t=teaspoon, T=tablespoon, w/=with, w/out = without

Regular Lunch Fuel (300-400 calories) cont.:

Taco Bell® **Bean Burrito** *or* Grilled Chicken Burrito

6" po-boy sandwich w/grilled seafood and red sauce (instead of tartar sauce)

Arby's*® **Junior Roast Beef Sandwich

***Sm burger** or ***cheeseburger** (such as *McDonald's*® kid's size or *Burger King® Mustard Whopper *Jr*® (w/mustard instead of mayo)

Hardee's*® **Hot Ham 'N' Cheese™ Sandwich

Super Lunch Fuel (500-600 calories):

Lg grilled chicken sandwich w/mayo or sauce or get it without sauce and have 10 french fries

Soup and sushi. Bowl of miso *or* egg drop soup and 10 pieces of sushi w/soy sauce, horseradish, & ginger

Pizza. 2 lg slices plain or onion/mushroom/ham pizza

12" Sub. 12" sub w/mustard or low-fat mayonnnaise or oil such as *Subway*® Veggie Delite, Turkey Breast, Ham, Roast Beef, *Subway* Club®, *Tuna or Seafood & Crab® made with light mayo

Restaurant grilled chicken salad (w/croutons & cheese) w/fat-free dressing (or 2T lowfat) & slice of bread or roll

Small *Gardenburger*® on bun (mustard, ketchup, lettuce, tomato, onion) with 20 french fries *or* the **Steak-size *Gardenburger*®** on large roll

Applebee's® **Chicken Fajita Quesadilla** or Lowfat **Lemon Chicken Pasta**

Boston Market®: **¼ roasted white meat chicken** (w/out skin or wing), corn, steamed vegetables, new potatoes

Fazoli's® **large spaghetti** with tomato or meat sauce

KFC® **Tender Roast Chicken sandwich** ("no sauce"), corn on the cob, BBQ baked beans

Wendy's® **Grilled Chicken Sandwich**, side salad w/reduced fat Italian dressing, & small bowl of chili

Wendy's® **plain baked potato** topped with small chili

***Sm burger or cheeseburger** (kid's size) w/mustard, ketchup *and* small fries

***Quarter pound burger** w/mustard, ketchup

c=cup, lg=large, med= medium, oz=ounce, sl=slice, sm=small, SW=sandwich, t=teaspoon, T=tablespoon, w/=with, w/out = without

Premium Lunch Fuel (700-800 calories):
Double any of the Regular Fuel choices

12" Sub w/low-fat mayonnnaise *or* oil such as *Subway*®
Veggie Delite, Turkey Breast, Ham, Roast Beef,
Subway Club®, *Tuna or *Seafood & Crab® made
w/light mayo plus small bag of fat-free chips or pretzels

Pizza. 2 large slices thick crust (or 3 slices thin crust)
onion/pepper/mushroom/ham pizza

Steak-size *Gardenburger*® on lg roll w/mustard, lettuce,
tomato, and onion plus 10 french fries

Large grilled chicken salad w/4T low-fat dressing
and lg yeast roll

***Boston Market*®: ¼ roasted white meat chicken**
(w/out skin or wing), corn, steamed vegetables, and
new potatoes, cornbread

***Lg grilled chicken** sw w/out mayo or sauce *and* 20
french fries

***Quarter pound burger** w/mustard, ketchup *and* 20
french fries

▶ **Dinner Choices:**

Regular Dinner Fuel (300-400 calories):
**3oz grilled chicken, fish, sirloin steak, *or* pork
tenderloin** w/sm baked potato (or ½c rice), 1 teaspoon
margarine, & steamed vegetables ("no butter")

**6oz grilled chicken, fish, sirloin steak, *or* pork
tenderloin** with steamed vegetables

Salad bar: 2c raw veggies, 2T chickpeas, 2T kidney
beans, and 3T fat-free dressing. Plus ½c fresh fruit,
and 2" square cornbread

1½c Chicken & vegetable stir-fry ("prepared with
very little oil") with ½c steamed rice

Pasta (1c) w/tomato sauce & 1 sm slice Italian bread

***Olive Garden*® Capellini Primavera** or Capellini
Pomodoro (luncheon portion)

***Mexican tacos:** 3oz chicken fajita meat, 2 tortillas,
lettuce, salsa

---

c=cup, lg=large, med= medium, oz=ounce, sl=slice, sm=small,
SW=sandwich, t=teaspoon, T=tablespoon, w/=with, w/out = without

Super Dinner Fuel (500-600 calories):

3oz grilled chicken, sirloin steak, pork tenderloin, *or* fish w/sm baked potato (or ½c rice), steamed vegetables ("no butter"), sm dinner roll, & 1 teaspoon margarine

6oz grilled chicken, fish, sirloin steak, *or* pork tenderloin w/sm baked potato (or ½c rice), steamed vegetables, & 1 teaspoon margarine

Salad bar: 2c raw veggies, 2T chickpeas, 2T kidney beans, & 3T fat-free dressing. ½c fresh fruit, 1 bowl broth-based soup, and cornbread (2"X3").

Chicken & vegetable stir-fry, 2c ("prepared with very little oil") & 1c steamed rice

1½c Pasta with tomato sauce, red or white clam sauce, *or* Bolognese sauce. Add slice of Italian bread if you chose the tomato sauce

***Olive Garden®* Capellini Primavera or Pomodoro,** luncheon portion & lightly buttered breadstick

Mexican tacos: 3 oz chicken fajita meat, 2 tortillas, lettuce, salsa plus ¾c Mexican rice *or* bean soup

Premium Dinner Fuel (700-800 calories):

4oz grilled chicken, sirloin steak, pork tenderloin, *or* fish w/sm baked potato (or ½c rice), & steamed broccoli ("no butter"), 2t margarine, & lg dinner roll

6oz grilled chicken, fish, sirloin steak, *or* pork tenderloin w/sm baked potato (or ½c rice), steamed vegetables, 1 large yeast roll, 2 teaspoons margarine

Salad bar: 2c raw veggies, 2T chickpeas, 2T kidney beans, & 3T fat-free dressing. ½c fresh fruit, 1 bowl broth-based soup, sm cornbread, & 1c frozen yogurt

Beef & vegetable stir-fry, 2c ("prepared with very little oil") w/1c steamed rice and fortune cookie

Pasta (2c) w/tomato, red clam sauce, or Bolognese sauce. Lightly buttered breadstick *or* 2sl Italian bread

***Olive Garden®* luncheon portion Capellini Primavera or Capellini Pomodoro,** bowl of Minestrone soup, and lightly buttered breadstick

Mexican tacos: 3oz chicken fajita meat, 2 tortillas, lettuce, salsa. ¾c Mexican rice & ¾c bean soup

---

c=cup, lg=large, med= medium, oz=ounce, sl=slice, sm=small, SW=sandwich, t=teaspoon, T=tablespoon, w/=with, w/out = without

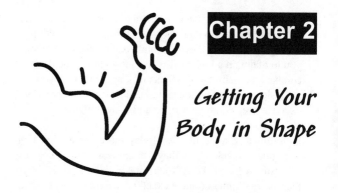

Chapter 2

*Getting Your
Body in Shape*

In This Chapter:
▶Exercise Essentials: what, when, & how
▶Fun Ways to Fit Exercise into a Busy Day
▶*Dr Jo's Hotel Room Workout*

If your car is involved in an accident, it's either repaired in the shop or, if it's totaled, you get a new car. When our body is in need of repair, fixing it is not quite that simple. This is the only body we'll ever get, so it's imperative to keep it in shape. But exercise isn't just for maintaining the outside in good physical shape, it keeps us healthy in the inside as well.

Did you know that the American Heart Association identified inactivity as a risk factor for heart disease – the number one killer? Other benefits of exercise include: control of blood glucose, maintenance of respiratory fitness, improved bone strength, reduced depression, and better sleep. According to research published in the Journal of Personality and Social Psychology, exercise was found to be the "most effective mood-regulating behavior" – better than many drugs! Exercise also helps you refocus, unwind after a long day, and bring out the creative juices by sparking the production of endorphins – mood-elevating brain chemicals. It also helps you to maintain a high energy level throughout the day and combats the debilitating effects of long hours of travel, altered sleep and eating schedules, and jet lag. In other words, exercise keeps both your mind and body in shape.

Unfortunately, a recent USA Today survey noted that 49% of frequent travelers said they were in worse shape because of business travel. USA Today stated that "travelers drop their normal fitness routine exactly when they most need its energizing effects."

Exercise Essentials

▶ **How Much & What Kind of Exercise Is Right for Me?**
The American College of Sports Medicine is the largest, most respected sports medicine and exercise science organization in the world. They recommend three types of exercise: aerobic activity to condition the heart and body, resistance training to strengthen muscles, and flexibility training for stretching.

Exercise Recommendations by ACSM*	
Aerobic Activity	20-60 minutes (in 10+ minute bouts) of walking, biking, swimming, skating, climbing, aerobic dance, etc. to be performed 3-6 days per week. Burns calories, shapes our body, & conditions the heart and lungs.
Resistance Training	One set (8-15 repetitions) exercises that condition major muscle groups 2-3 days per week. Enhances strength, muscular endurance, & muscle mass.
Flexibility Training	Stretching major muscle groups 2-3 days a week. Important for maintaining a healthy range of motion, preventing injury, & reducing muscle soreness.

*The American College of Sports Medicine (www.acsm.org)

▶ **There are No Excuses.** If you're not currently exercising on a regular basis and receiving the health benefit, it's time to ask yourself why.

- **No time?** New research supports that your "workout" can be just as effective if you split it into 10 minute chunks. So skip the airport tram and take a brisk walk to the next terminal. You do have your luggage on wheels, right? Keep in mind, that although exercise "takes" time, it also "gives back" time through better health, improved sleep, and increased energy.

- **Too much to do?** Next time you're "stuck" on how to handle a situation or respond to that email, take a walk with a mini notepad and pen. Many people find that exercise has a way of stimulating creative and useful thoughts and solutions. Walking is a great forum for practicing your upcoming speech or your script to ask for a raise.

- **No workout room in the hotel or bad equipment?** Check with the concierge. There's probably a workout facility in town that will give you a discount just by showing your hotel room key. Or try *Dr Jo's Hotel Room Workout* at the end of this chapter.

- **Bad weather outside?** Book a hotel that's close to a mall; they're often open longer hours to accommodate mall walkers. Or walk the halls of the hotel in the evening to decrease stress and walk off dinner. Fit in a "stair stepper" routine by walking up and down a safe stair well.

- **Exhausted?** Most of us aren't tired due to strenuous physical work. Chances are it's mental stress that's zapping our energy – and exercise is just what we need to recharge our body and mind. Find some movement that you really like and get going. You'll be happy you did.

- **No motivation?** Call 800-YOUR-BODY for three free minutes of fitness counseling (8am-5pm PST) from The Aerobic and Fitness Association of America (www.afaa.com). Or log onto www.fitnesslink.com for self-help quizzes, exercises, and tips for getting in shape.

How to Stay Healthy & Fit on the Road

- **No weights?** Pack your tubing (stretchy giant rubber bands), *AquaBells* (lightweight, collapsible forms that you fill with water at your destination), or *Xertubes*™ (rubber tubes with handles). I use the *Xertubes*™ when I'm on the road; they're easy to pack and provide a great workout.

- **Too stressful?** If you find exercise stressful, you're probably working out at too high of an intensity or your workout is too long. Beginners should start slowly with just ten minutes of aerobic exercise and increase the length by no more than 10% a week (11 minutes for week two, 12 minutes for week three, etc). Working out will often feel stressful if you don't like the activity – keep looking for an option you enjoy.

- **Bored?** Don't just exercise. Pair your workout with a book, newspaper, or magazine. Motivate yourself by allowing yourself to read your leisure book only when you're exercising. Listen to TV, books-on-tape, or music (www.sportsmusic.com has music to fit your pace). You can buy audiotapes at bookstores and second hand stores, borrow them from the local library, or rent them from grocery stores. When you're traveling, rent tapes at *Cracker Barrel*® restaurants. They will charge full sales price for the audio tape and refund all but $3 per week when you return the tape to *any* of their locations.

- **Don't know what to do?** Get a trainer. Larger facilities and health resorts can often help you schedule a personal fitness trainer or call AFAA at 800-YOUR-BODY for a referral in your area. Exercise videos can also teach you what to do. The hotel fitness facility may have some exercise videos or bring your own. You can find hundreds of exercise videos (and reviews) at www.collagevideo.com. Once you become familiar with your routine, connect your VCR at home to any stereo system with a tape deck. This allows you to transform your exercise video into a portable audio workout for travel.

Fun Ways to Fit Exercise into a Busy Day

▶ **How to Get into the Exercise Habit.** Exercise should be consistent, pleasurable, help you meet your goals, and adaptable to your ever-changing schedule. The following strategies will improve your odds of success:

- **Make it a priority.** There's no excuse not to exercise if it's high enough on your priority list.

- **Set a goal.** Sign up for a 10K run, a coed soccer team, or a fund-raising bike ride. You'll have more of an incentive to work out when you're on the road.

- **Just say NO.** Learn to say "no" to unwanted and unnecessary tasks and obligations that take you away from exercising. When you find yourself distracted away from exercise, ask yourself: "Is what I am doing or about to be doing leading me towards my goal?"

- **Set aside a specific time each day.** There's no best time of the day to exercise – it's whatever works best for you. What's important is to schedule your exercise. Put it into your daily calendar or it will be too easy to fill your day with other things.

- **Do it first.** If your energy wanes as the day goes on, exercise first thing in the morning or as soon as you check into your hotel.

- **Do it just before you return home.** Has this ever happened? You've checked out of your room that morning, completed your business, and still have a few hours before your flight? Consider asking if you can return to last night's hotel to use the exercise facilities and shower. There's a good chance they'll let you.

- **Make it easy and regular.** The American Heart Association points out that with just five weeks of inactivity, individuals lose 50% of their fitness ability. So skipping exercise for a week or two will make it that much more difficult when you get back on a regular schedule. Find an exercise routine that is easy enough for you to do on a regular basis.

51

- **Get rid of the "all or nothing" mindset.** When you don't have time for your usual workout, don't skip it entirely. Do ten minutes in the morning, ten minutes at noon, and ten minutes at night. You'll get the same benefits as a full 30 minute workout.

- **Have an alternate plan.** I had a friend who swam during his lunch hour. But when he developed bursitis in his shoulder, he stopped exercising all together. Your body will be stronger and healthier if you cross-train with more than one type of aerobic activity. And you'll be more likely to stay in shape because you can be flexible with your routine. No pool? Get on the exercise bike. Treadmill's broken? Go for a walk. Too cold for a walk outside? Take it indoors. No time for a walk? Just do some sit-ups, push-ups, and stretching. What's your Plan B?

▶ **Where to Workout.** With just a few items of clothing (see the *Getting Your Wheels in Gear* chapter), you will be ready to workout. Where?

- **Everywhere!** Pack your sneakers in your briefcase. At work, take the stairs instead of the elevator. When you need to run an errand during the day, slip on your sneakers, and step out at a brisk pace. Take a walk during your lunch break or when you need to de-stress. In the evenings, take a walk in the convention area.

- **In the hotel workout room.** The American Hotel and Motel Association, estimates that about 40% of US hotels have some kind of fitness facility. If you are more likely to exercise if a gym is available on-site, be sure to ask about their fitness facilities when making reservations. Don't just ask if they have a fitness club, ask what working equipment they have, the hours (incredible as it seems, some are only open during business hours), or if they have arrangements with local health clubs. You may also want to know if they have a heated pool or aerobic classes.

- **In your hotel room.** Some hotels have an in-room exercise treadmill, Nordic track, health rider, stair stepper, or bike. Or (for free or a fee) will offer to bring one up to your room. But don't always believe the computer readouts on the exercise equipment. The number of calories burned tend to be overestimated by 10-30%. Or do *Dr Jo's Hotel Room Workout* which is detailed at the end of this chapter.

- **At a nearby fitness club.** Although there may be plenty of fitness clubs in the area, you'll often pay less when you take advantage of your hometown health club associations around the world. For example, YMCA has an "AWAY" (Always Welcome at the Y) program which admits a member to most YMCA facilities for free or a small fee. Over 3500 other clubs are affiliated with the nonprofit association International Health and Racquet Sportsclub Association (IHRSA) whose Passport Program grants reciprocal guest privileges in some 50 countries, usually at a minimal fee. With an All-Club membership at a 24 hour Fitness or Q Sport Club, you can visit any of their locations in the US or abroad at no charge for up to 30 days.

- **Outside.** Even if you're traveling for business, explore the city on foot or walk between appointments. Go for a walk, run around the local park, jump rope in the pool area, or just run around the hotel a few dozen times.

- **In your seat.** OK, so you can't do aerobics while in a car, bus, or airline seat. But, you can take a few minutes every hour to stretch and keep your body limber - don't do these while you're driving. Hold each stretch for 20 seconds. Try these: neck stretches (tilt your head to each side and hold; then drop your chin to your chest and hold), chest stretch (grasp hands behind neck and press elbows back), shoulder stretch (keeping your arm straight, extend it across the chest and use the other hand to pull it in; repeat to the other side), and knee kiss (one at a time, pull each leg to your chest, grasp with both hands, and hold). Add a few, slow shoulder rolls and ankle rolls in each direction.

- **In the aisle or at a rest area.** Try these stretches for 20 seconds: calf stretch (place hands on car or wall; move one leg two feet back and stretch, repeat with other leg), quad stretch (holding onto wall, bend one knee and grasp ankle, repeat with the other leg), back stretch (holding onto pole or seat, squat down, and lean forward slightly), and hamstring stretch (with leg outstretched, place heel on short wall).

- **At the airport.** Check your bags in an airport locker for a half-hour and walk around the airport. Or if all your bags are on wheels (and why aren't they?), you can pull them along. Or take a cab to a nearby mall. The Mall of America in Minneapolis has large luggage lockers to store your luggage while you walk.

- **Near the airport.** If you have a long layover at an airport, take a break from the food court and work out. While a few airports have a health and fitness facility on premise, many more are just a walk or short drive away. The clubs on the following pages are just some of the possibilities. Each location offers a day pass (usually $5-15, but may be as high as $25) for travelers and may offer a discount for showing your airline ticket.

Long Airport Layover? Where to Workout:

Atlanta (Hartsfield-Atlanta Int'l) – 1. Attractive Bodies Health & Fitness Club (770-997-2339, 5466 Crestridge Dr, Atlanta, GA 30349) is a 5-minute ride. 2. Fitness Plus (770-994-9595, 6326 HW 85, Riverdale, GA 30274) is a 10-minute taxi ride.

Baltimore/Washington Int'l – take the free 1-mile hotel shuttle to BWI Marriot (410-859-8300).

Boston (Logan Int'l) – Airport Hilton Hotel (617-568-6882) has complimentary hotel shuttle.

Charlotte (Charlotte/Douglas Int'l) – Gold's Gym (704-554-1010, 6010 Fairview Road, Charlotte, NC 28210) is a 10-minute taxi ride.

Airport Workouts (continued):

Chicago (Midway) – 1-mile cab ride to Al's Gym (708-563-9334, 5301 W 65ᵗʰ St, Chicago, IL 60638).

Chicago (O'Hare) – The Athletic Club at the Hilton Chicago O'Hare Airport (773-601-1723) is accessible through underground tunnel.

Cincinnati (Greater Cincinnati/Northern Kentucky Int'l) – Fitworks Fitness & Sports Therapy (859-282-0600, 7541 Mall Rd, Florence, KY 41042) is a 10-minute taxi ride.

Cleveland (Cleveland Hopkins Int'l Airport) – Bally Total Fitness (216-267-3500, 14571 Snow Rd, Brookpark, OH 44142) is 10 minutes away.

Dallas (DFW) – 1. Athletic and Tennis Club, Hilton DFW Lakes (817-481-6647, 1800 Highway 26E, Grapevine, TX, 76051) is 10 minutes away. Take a cab or Hilton shuttle. 2. Irving Fitness (972-257-0221, 3909 West Airport Freeway, Irving, TX 75062) is 15 minutes away in opposite direction.

Denver Int'l – 1. World Gym (303-344-4413, 543 Sable Blvd, Aurora, CO 80011) is 15-20 minutes SW of airport. 2. Stapleton Fitness Center (303-329-2777) in the Radisson Hotel (303-321-3500, 3333 Quebec St, Denver, CO 80207) is about 30 minutes W.

Detroit (Detroit Metro) – 10 minutes away is Wayne Racquet & Exercise Club (734-728-2900, 4635 Howe Road, Wayne, MI 48184).

Ft Lauderdale (Fort Lauderdale/Hollywood Int'l) - Gold's Gym (954-927-3481, 3120 Oakwood Blvd, Hollywood, FL 33020) is a 6-minute cab ride.

Honolulu Int'l – Gold's Gym (808-533-7111, 768 South St, Honolulu, HI 96813) is a 10-minute drive.

Houston (Hobby) – Bally's Total Fitness (713-941-3584, 1418 Spencer Hwy, Pasadena, TX 77587) is a 10-15 minute taxi ride.

Airport Workouts (continued):

Houston (Intercontinental) – Take 15-minute taxi ride or free Wyndham Greenspoint shuttle. Greenspoint Club is behind the Wyndham on 5th floor of parking garage (281-875-0191, 16925 N. Chase, Houston, TX 77060). Clothing available.

Indianapolis Int'l – Excel Fitness is just 5 minutes away (317-244-3500, 6450 W10^{th} St, Indianapolis, IN 46214)

Irvine, CA (John Wayne) – Less than 5 minutes away is 24 Hour Fitness (949-250-4422, 18007 Von Karman Ave, Irvine, CA 92612).

Kansas City Int'l – Just Total Fitness (816-505-0900, 8114 NW Prairie View Rd, Kansas City, MO 64151) is 10 minutes away.

Las Vegas (McCarran Int'l) – located on the 2nd floor right above baggage claim is 24 Hour Fitness (702-261-3971). For $15 extra you get (for keeps) shorts, T-shirt, socks, and towel. Rental shoes also available.

Los Angeles (LAX) – Walk the mile or take Hilton shuttle to 24 Hour Fitness/LAX Hilton (310-410-9909).

Memphis Int'l – Take a 5-minute cab ride to Fitness Plus (901-345-1036, 2598 Corporate Ave E., Memphis, TN 38132).

Miami – Health Club at the Miami Int'l Airport Hotel (305-871-4100) is located in Concourse E, 2nd level.

Minneapolis-St. Paul Int'l – Appletree Fitness Center is 10 minutes away on 3rd floor of the Holiday Inn Select (952-854-3691, 3 Appletree Square, Minn., MN 55425).

Nashville Int'l – Gold's Gym is a 5-minute cab ride (615-366-1063, 2311 Murfreesboro Rd, Nashville, TN 37217).

Newark Int'l – Airport Hilton is just across the highway, but allow 10-15 minutes. (908-351-3900, 1170 Spring St, Newark, NJ 07201).

Airport Workouts (continued):

New Orleans Int'l – Curetons Sports Club is 5-10 minutes away (504-466-7642, 1712 Vegas Drive, Metairie, LA 70003).

New York (John F. Kennedy Int'l) – Cross Island Sports & Fitness Center Inc is a 5-10 minute taxi ride (718-528-7592, 21910 South Conduit Avenue, Springfield Gardens, NY 11413).

New York (La Guardia) – La Guardia Marriot Hotel's health club is located in their lower lobby (718-565-8900 X 6519) 2 minutes away; call for courtesy shuttle.

Orlando Int'l – World Gym is 5-10 minutes away (407-249-5506, 1900 Century Plaza, S. Semoran Blvd, Orlando, FL 32812).

Philadelphia Int'l – Sports Club is a 15-minute drive (610-833-2000, MacDade & Fairview Rd, Woodlyn, PA 19094).

Phoenix (Sky Harbor Int'l) – Arizona Athletic Club is a 5-minute taxi ride (480-894-2281, 1425 W 14th St., Tempe, AZ 85281).

Pittsburgh Int'l – Airport Fitness Pittsburgh (412-472-5231) is just inside the terminal. Workout clothing rental is available for an extra fee.

Portland Int'l – Nelsons Nautilus (503-254-7710, 8333 Northeast Russell Street, Portland, OR 97220) is 5-10 minutes away.

Salt Lake City Int'l – 1. Metro Sports Club (801-364-8803, ZCMI Center Mall, SLC, UT 84101) is 5-10 minutes away downtown. 2. The Firm (801-328-2639, 324 S. State St, SLC, UT 84111) is also downtown and open longer hours than Metro.

San Antonio Int'l – Olympic Gym (210-829-5040, 8611 North New Braunfels Avenue, San Antonio, TX 78217) is a 5-minute drive.

Airport Workouts (continued):

San Diego Int'l – The health club is located in the East Tower of the Sheraton San Diego Hotel & Marina (619-291-2900, 1590 Harbor Island Drive, San Diego, CA 92101). Free 2-3 minute hotel shuttle.

San Francisco Int'l – Gold's Gym (415-552-4653, 1001 Brannan St, San Francisco, CA 94103) is 15-20 minutes away.

San Jose Int'l – Gold's Gym (408-988-4494, 1900 Duane Ave, San Jose, CA 95054) is a 5-10 minute taxi ride.

St. Louis (Lambert-St. Louis Int'l) – 1. St. Louis Workout (314-633-3020, 212 North Kings Highway Boulevard, Saint Louis, MO 63108). 2. Westport

Tampa Int'l – Beach Park Health Club (813-839-4444, 3637 South Manhattan Avenue, Tampa, FL 33629) is 10-15 minutes away.

Tucson Int'l – Mid-Valley Athletic Club (520-792-3654, 140 South Tucson Boulevard, Tucson, AZ 85716) is a 10-minute taxi ride

Washington DC (Washington Nat'l) – 1. Crystal Gateway Sport & Health (703-416-4900, 1235 Jefferson-Davis Highway, Arlington, VA 22202). 2. Crystal Park Sport & Health (703-486-3380, 2231 Crystal Drive, Arlington, VA 22202). Both (offering different amenities) are near each other and a 5-minute cab ride.

▶ **Where to Find Walk/Run Courses around Town.** There are some very beautiful walks/runs in just about every city all over the world. These include the 7 mile river walk in Columbus, Georgia, the 185 mile Chesapeake and Ohio Canal running from Washington DC to Cumberland, MD, and the Historic walk around Old Sacramento and the State House Gardens. Where can you find out about these areas?

- **Concierge.** They usually know where there's a safe park and will often have an actual running/walking map.

- **Convention & Visitor's Bureau.** Drop by or call ahead to ask for information on parks and recreation facilities as well as self-guided walking or cycling tours in the area. You'll find US offices at www.towd.com and international bureaus at www.officialtravelinfo.com.

- **American Running Association.** (1-800-776-2732, www.AmericanRunning.org). You don't have to be a runner to join this group started by the Surgeon General back in 1968 – walkers are welcome. In addition to a monthly newsletter, the $25/year membership (just $15 if you mention that you heard about them in this book) allows you access to medical and fitness experts to answer your questions. Online, you'll find hundreds of free running maps for cities all over the world. The maps were started by an airline pilot and are constantly being updated by runners.

- **Runner's World.** (www.runnersworld.com/ontheroad.home.html) These articles share running courses, fitness clubs, and races all over the world.

- **American Volkssport Association (AVA).** (210-659-2112). AVA is a nonprofit national organization dedicated to promoting the benefits of health and physical fitness for people of all ages. Events are open to everyone but annual membership (including bimonthly newsletter) is $20 per individual or $25 for a family (you'll get $5 off membership by mentioning that you read about them in this book). AVA sponsors organized weekend walks (usually 5K-20K). In addition, local groups maintain over 1000 walks to do whenever you want. Details are in their book *Starting Point: AVA's Guide to 1272 Trails in America*, $10.95) which describes where to pick up local maps and details of where to walk. Call 800-830-WALK to hear about walking, biking, and swimming events in every state.

- **American Hiking Society** (AHS). AHS provides a wealth of hiking and trail resources including discounts on selected maps and guide books. The $25 annual membership includes access to AHS's 120 member clubs. (301-565-6704, email: amhiker@aol.com).

▶ **Other Options for Exercise**

- **Take in a game.** Resort hotels, if convenient to your business and within your budget, often offer tennis or golf. Since airlines offer the best flight rates when you stay over a Saturday night, your boss may agree to pay for a weekend stay so you can play.

- **Find a partner anywhere.** Search for a partner for running, tennis, golf, or a hike (a free service) at www.SportsMatchOnLine.com.

- **Go for a swim.** Swimming is a great toner and can be very relaxing. If the hotel pool is too small to swim laps, go water jogging or simply tread water in the deep end. Need some music? Check out *Speedo®*'s waterproof radio. No pool in your hotel? Search by state at http://lornet.com/SGOL for a list of year round, public and private, lap swimming pools that admit visitors for free or at a day rate. Listing includes name, phone number, pool size, cost, directions, and maps.

- **Get adventurous**. Search the internet for "outdoor adventure" and get a long list of associations, activities, and tours around the country. Or check your destination's newspaper or online city guide for scheduled hikes or other outdoor excursions.

- **Have a "working out lunch."** Instead of a working business lunch or a business discussion over drinks, opt for a "working-out" lunch where you discuss business while walking or working out on exercise equipment. This has three benefits: gives you a workout, cuts down on opportunities to overeat or overdrink, and builds a bond with the other person or people.

- **Get jumping.** Bring along a jump rope for a quick and easy way to get the heart pumping. If you ever forget your rope, try "make-believe" jump rope. It's harder than you think. If there's a hotel room below yours, it's best to take the workout outside or to the pool deck.

- **Go skating.** Roller or ice skating is good exercise. To find a roller skating rink in your city, log onto www.rollerskate.net or www.frogsonice.com/skateweb/clubs.html for an ice skating rink.

- **Have a ball.** Golf courses all over the world can be found at http://course.golfweb.com and squash courts at www.squashtalk.

Dr Jo's Hotel Room Workout

My husband, a former Marine officer, was stationed on a Navy ship for an extended period of time in the Far East. Feeling the adverse combination of a sedentary lifestyle and the high caloric Navy diet, he developed a 45 minute strength and endurance routine he could do in the available closet-size space. More than two decades later, he still uses this exact regimen at home and in hotel rooms when he can't get to the gym.

I've since improved upon his routine to create *Dr Jo's Hotel Room Workout.* This is an all-in-one complete body work-out that meets ACSM requirements (I consulted with speaker/exercise physiologist, Karen Behrend, MEd) to strengthen, condition, and stretch your body safely in a lim-ited space. Three variations are offered for different levels of fitness. The 1st Gear Program is a 30-minute beginner work-out, 2nd Gear is a 40-minute fitness routine, and 3rd Gear is a 50-minute advanced workout.

Dr Jo's Hotel Room Workout* At a Glance			
	1st Gear (30 min)	2nd Gear (40 min)	3rd Gear (50 min)
▶ Warm Up (Jogging or marching in place):			
	3 min	3 min	3 min
▶ Circuit Training (alternate until you complete 8 sets of each):			
Aerobic	1 min	2 min	3 min
Strengthening	8-15 reps	10-20 reps	15-25 reps
▶ Cool Down:			
Slow Moves	1-2 min	1-2 min	1-2 min
Stomach Crunches	8-15 reps	10-20 reps	15-25 reps
Flexibility	8 stretches	8 stretches	8 stretches
*Workout is shown at three levels affecting both time & intensity. 1st Gear is for beginners, 2nd Gear is for the intermediate, and 3rd Gear is for the avid athlete.			

▶ **Service Recommendations**

- **Check with your doctor first** as with any workout program.
- **The no-pain/no-gain mentality is NOT a healthy mindset.** A proper workout should not leave you feeling totally exhausted.
- **Monitor your heart rate** throughout the Circuit Training phase. Place your fingers on the radial artery which is located at the palm side of the wrist near the base of the thumb. Count your pulse for a 10-second period and compare to the chart to the right. As an example, a 45 year old person should maintain their pulse between 16 and 24

Training Heart Rate Zone	
Age	Heart Rate* (per 10 seconds)
20-29	18-28
30-39	17-26
40-49	16-24
50-59	15-23
60-69	14-22
70-79	13-20
80-89	12-19
90+	12-18
*Based on theoretical maximum heart rate (220-age) multiplied by a training range of 55-85%.	

beats per 10 second period.

- **Use common sense.** If the intensity feels too difficult, slow down the pace to a more comfortable level. If you experience symptoms such as dizziness, nausea or chest pains, stop the exercise session immediately and consult your physician.

- **Do the toning exercises very slowly** – about 2-4 seconds in each direction.

- **Remember to advance slowly** from beginner movements to more advanced. And feel free to adapt the workout routine to meet your special needs.

- **Get yourself an** *Xertube™* for the resistance exercises. These lightweight, inexpensive, and easy-to-pack resistance tubes are available in five color-coded resistances from the very light to the ultra. Order from my website at www.DrJo.com or contact Spri direct (www.spriproducts.com, 800-222-7774). Spri also has jump ropes and other helpful exercise equipment and resources.

▶ **Warm-Up (3 minutes).** This phase of the workout helps to prepare your body for exercise by increasing blood circulation to the muscles, preventing injury to the body, and reducing muscle soreness. Start off slowly with 3 minutes of marching, jogging in place, or just dancing to the music.

> 1st Gear: lift your feet slightly off the floor
> 2nd Gear: bring feet 6-12" off the floor
> 3rd Gear: bring your knee parallel to waist
>   in a brisk march or jog in place

Although stretching *after* a workout is critical to prevent strains, sprains, and muscle soreness, it's not necessary to stretch *before* exercise – but go ahead and do some stretches now if you want to.

How to Stay Healthy & Fit on the Road

▶ **Circuit Training** – Complete eight sets of aerobic exercise alternating with one set of each of the eight strengthening exercises.

- **Aerobic exercise** – Adjusting the intensity according to your fitness level, choose from any of the following: jump rope, march in place, twist (remember the dance

1st Gear: 1 minute	
2nd Gear: 2 minutes	
3rd Gear: 3 minutes	

  Chubby Checkers made famous?), run in place, or just dance! Practice some of the moves from an aerobics class, like the grapevine. Make believe you're skiing – keep both feet together and jump from side to side. Or like a pendulum, swing one leg out to the side, as it comes back in to the middle, kick the other leg out. The important thing is to get your pulse up and have fun!

- **Strengthening exercises** – After each set of aerobic exercise, do one of the following strengthening exercises. Using an

1st Gear: 8-15 repetitions (reps)	
2nd Gear: 10-20 reps	
3rd Gear: 15-25 reps	

  Xertube™, make sure the movements are done slowly (2-4 seconds in each direction). Control the tube at all times; do not let it spring back. Keep your abdominals tight throughout the exercises.

1. Squats – anchor tube under both feet (about shoulder width apart). Hold handles at shoulders, elbows open with tubing behind body. Sit back slowly until knees are approximately parallel to the floor. Make sure that your knees do not go over your toes.

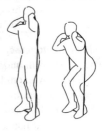

Start   Finish

2. Lunges – wrap middle of tube around one foot and hold handles at shoulder height in front of your body. Place other leg approximately two feet back. With weight predominately on the front foot, flex both knees until front upper leg is approximately parallel to the floor. Do recommended reps; repeat with the other leg.

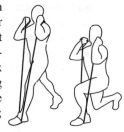

Start   Finish

3. Hamstring curls – thread one end of tube through the other to make a loop. Place loop around your right ankle and hold tube handle in the left hand. Step on the tube so that your right toe is pointed to the ground, but can go no higher. Pull your right heel slowly towards your buttocks and return. After the recommended reps, repeat with your left leg.

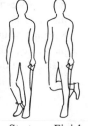

Start   Finish

4. Push-ups – just like you remember from your phys ed classes. Lay on your belly and place your hands under your shoulders. Do your push ups on your toes or knees.

5. Seated row – sit on the floor with legs straight out. Wrap the tube around your feet by placing the middle of the tube over the tops of your feet, wrap it around the outsides, and pull the ends between your feet. Grasp the handles with an overhand hold. In one movement, flex elbows and twist forearms to finish with palms facing up and little fingers at your lowest ribs.

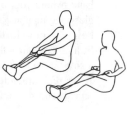

Start   Finish

65

6. Side lateral raise – stand with feet positioned hip width apart with tube anchored under both feet. Use overhand grip and place hands on the side of body. Keeping arms straight, lift until elbows reach shoulder height.

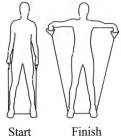

Start   Finish

7. Bicep curls – in the same position as the side lateral raise, place hands in front of the body in a underhand grip. Keeping your upper arms in place, flex elbows until hands reach shoulder height.

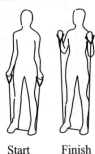

Start   Finish

8. Tricep overhead extension – hold tube handle in left hand. Lift arm up and bend at elbow. Keeping elbow pointing to ceiling, let tube fall behind you. Place right hand behind your back and grasp the tube about a foot below your left hand. Straighten your left arm to a soft elbow lock position. After recommended reps, repeat with the right arm.

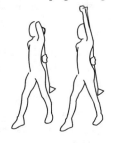

Start   Finish

▶ **Cooldown, Abs, & Flexibility Moves**

- **Slow moves.** March in place (with low knees) or walk the room until heart rate drops below your training heart rate zone (1-2 min).

- **Stomach crunches.** Lie on floor with bent knees. Raise head and upper body slightly and do three sets of stomach crunches: one forward and one set to each side.

  | 1st Gear: 8-15 reps |
  | 2nd Gear: 10-20 reps |
  | 3rd Gear: 15-25 reps |

- **Flexibility moves** - hold each movement for 10-20 seconds and do not bounce. Stretch the least flexible extremity first:

1. Calf stretch. Standing up, face a wall with feet about a foot away and hands against the wall directly across from shoulders. Extend one leg about two feet back and hold. Repeat with other leg.

2. Side stretch. Sit up straight with legs apart in a straddle position. Stretch forward from the hips, hold. Repeat to each side.

3. Inner thigh stretch. Sit up straight with bottoms of feet together. Hold ankles and lean forward from the hips.

4. Pretzel. Sit straight up with bent knees and ankles crossed. Cross one foot over the other knee. Twisting your body slightly in the direction of the upright knee, hug it and hold.

5. Double knee hold. Lie on back and hug both knees to your chest.

6. Hamstring stretch. Lie on back with feet flat on the floor and knees bent. Extend one leg, slightly bent, and pull gently towards your chest. Repeat with the other leg.

7. Quad stretch. Lie on one side. Bend the top knee and grasp ankle keeping knees together. Repeat to the other side.

8. Shoulder stretch. Gently pull elbow across the chest to the opposite shoulder using the other hand.

Congratulations. You're done!

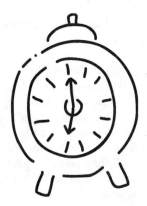

Chapter 3

Setting The Snooze Control

In This Chapter:
▶ Are You Getting Enough Sleep?
▶ Tips to Help You Get Your Zzzzzs
▶ *Dr Jo's D.R.E.A.M. Formula*
▶ Recharge Your Batteries with a PowerNap

In today's fast-paced business environment, the expression, "if you snooze, you lose" is often valid. But if you take the expression literally and forfeit the sleep you need, you risk losing even more. Sleep deprivation can kill. The US National Highway Traffic Safety Administration estimates that approximately 100,000 police-reported crashes each year involve drowsiness or fatigue as a principal causal factor. There are even some preliminary studies to suggest that long-term sleep debt could play a role in diabetes, obesity, breast cancer, and a weakened immune system resulting in more colds and other infections.

Lastly, sleep deprivation results in irritability, lack of concentration, impaired memory, poor judgement, and more fatigue-related errors. According to a recent article in the Baltimore Sun, former President Clinton was quoted as having said that "Every important mistake I've made in my life, I've made because I was tired."

Are You Getting Enough Sleep?

The National Sleep Foundation (NSF) says you're not. Their survey conducted in the year 2000 reports that adults sleep about an hour less than the eight hours recommended by sleep experts. In addition, nearly two-thirds of adults in the US expereienced insomnia at least a few nights per week during the past year. This includes being awake a lot during the night, difficulty falling asleep or waking up too early, and not being able to get back to sleep.

▶ **You're Getting Enough Zzzzs if…**
- You wake up naturally without an alarm clock
- You sleep the same amount of time on days off as on workdays
- You feel alert during the day even when driving or attending boring meetings

▶ **It's Not Just the Hours That Count.** We also require uninterrupted sleep. Our body's need to sleep is regulated by an internal clock or circadian rhythm. Sleep consists of repetitive and continuous cycles lasting approximately 90 minutes each. Each cycle begins with a light sleep state (kind of a "twilight zone") where your muscles relax. Then you progress through deeper stages of sleep that are considered to be critical for restoring both your physical and mental capacities. After an hour or so into the cycle, you shift into the highly active, dream-state characterized by rapid eye movements (REM sleep). The cycle then repeats itself again, but as the night goes on, the deep sleep states get shorter and the REM periods tend to become longer. Combined with this sleep-wake cycle, temperature variation and hormone secretion also play a role in the cycle. Your body temperature drops towards bedtime and the hormone, melatonin, rises (and peaks at midnight).

As tempting as it is to cut back on sleep to get work done, to spend time with family and friends, watch TV, log on the internet, or to work around the house before heading out of town, it's time to realize that the implications just aren't worth it. We lose more than we gain by depriving ourselves of sleep. Stop thinking of sleep as a wasteful activity, it's the way we recharge our batteries for our next day's performance.

Tips to Help You Get Your Zzzzzs

▶ **Watch What You Eat and Drink.**

• **Avoid caffeine in the afternoon and evening.** Most of us view caffeine as an instant pick-me-up, something to keep us going when we feel like we're running out of fuel. While caffeine *can* revive us, the effects of caffeine can linger for many hours – long after you need it. If you have a hard time sleeping, avoid caffeine for at least four to five hours before bedtime. Some people are even more sensitive and might have to skip caffeine after lunch. If you're tired when driving in the late evening, you may be better served to pull over to power nap instead of having a cup of coffee. It's recommended to limit caffeine to less than 200 mg per day and use medicinally – when you really need the effect. As you can see in this chart, coffee isn't the only source of caffeine:

Caffeine (mg) Content of Beverages, Foods, & Medicines	
Coffee: brewed (8oz)	100
Gourmet (8oz)	150
Decaffeinated (8oz)	5
Expresso (1)	35
Latte, cappucino, mocha (8oz)	35
Tea: brewed (8oz)	50
Iced (12 oz. glass)	70
Sodas: Those which list "caffeine" in the ingredient list including colas, Mello Yello, Big Red, Mountain Dew	50

continued on the next page

Caffeine (mg) Content of Beverages, Foods, & Medicines (cont.)	
Chocolate: Chocolate milk (1oz)	5
Dark chocolate (1oz)	20
Cocoa, chocolate milk (8 oz)	5
Chocolate-flavored syrup (1 oz)	5
Medicines: BC® powder (1 dose)	33
Anacin (2 tablet dose)	64
Midol (2 tablet dose)	120
Extra Strength Exedrin (2 tablet dose)	130
No Doz (1 tablet) or Vivarin (1 tablet)	200

- **Skip the night cap.** Alcohol may produce an initial sleepy effect, but it actually disrupts your sleep cycle. It increases the number of times you awaken in the later half of the night.

- **Cut back on the fluids.** Drinking too much of *any* beverage can lead to more awakenings because of the need to urinate during the night - especially as we get older. Drink plenty of fluids in the day and try to restrict your fluids before bedtime.

- **Avoid heartburn.** Heartburn is caused by acid and other stomach contents backing up into the esophagus. Lying down intensifies the heartburn; the pain can be severe enough to keep you awake. Common culprits for heartburn include foods such as tomato products, citrus fruits and juices, coffee (regular and decaffeinated), chocolate, peppermint, alcohol, fried foods, and other fatty foods. Some people also find spicy foods and carbonated beverages to cause some discomfort.

- **Calm down with the carbs.** Research indicates that carbohydrates release serotonin, a brain neurotransmitter, that makes you feel relaxed. So eat your protein (meat, eggs, cheese) during breakfast and lunch and eat a high carbohydrate, vegetarian evening meal (potatoes, pasta, cereal, rice, bread, vegetables, fruits). Some people stay away from sugar in the evening thinking it is a stimulant, but there isn't any research to back it up.

However, excess chocolate, especially dark chocolate, can provide a substantial caffeine boost.

- **Don't stuff yourself in the evening hours.** Eating too much of any food can make sleep difficult. A heavy meal close to bedtime may make you less comfortable when you settle down for your night's rest.

- **Don't go to bed hungry either.** Going to bed hungry can be as disruptive as going to bed too full. If your frequently have problems sleeping because your stomach is growling or you wake up in the middle of the night hungry, plan on a light dinner and have a bedtime snack.

- **Check your nutritional status**. If you suffer from restless leg syndrome – an urge to move the legs, often accompanied by creeping, crawling, or tingling sensation, ask your doctor for help. Iron deficiency or a need for more vitamin E seems to be responsible for some cases.

▶ **Avoid Stimulants.** Don't give yourself a "jumpstart" just before bedtime. Consider these:

- **Quit tobacco.** Nicotine, like caffeine, is a stimulant. Research has demonstrated that nicotine can cause difficulty in falling asleep and contribute to problems waking up. Smokers may also experience more nightmares. While giving up tobacco products may cause more sleep problems at first, the long-term effect on sleep – and your health – is worth it.

- **Check your medicine box.** You may be surprised to learn how many medications have a stimulating effect, including decongestants, antidepressants such as *Prozac*, and overmedication with thyroid hormones. Ask your doctor or pharmacist.

- **Exercise….just not right before bedtime.** People who exercise on a regular basis get to sleep faster and sleep deeper. Be patient, in one research study it took up to eight weeks of regular exercise for the effect to take place. But strenuous exercise right before bedtime raises your body temperature and may make you feel more alert. If it does, exercise in the morning or at least three hours before bedtime. (Exercise leads to a rise in body temperature with a corresponding fall in temperature five to six hours later – which then makes sleep easier). If there's no time to exercise earlier in the day, consider getting in just a light workout before bedtime.

▶ **Control Your Environment.** Some of our sleep problems are due to the fact that many of us have a natural circadian rhythm that is actually closer to 25 hours than 24. In order to keep ourselves aligned with the external 24 hour world, we need cues called Zeitgebers to reset our internal clock. Light is one of the most powerful regulators, but there are others that will be discussed later.

- **Keep the room dark.** Bright light can awaken you and throw off your internal clock. Make the room as dark as possible by turning off the bathroom light and closing the window covering completely. Pack a couple of clothes pins to keep it shut. If the light from under the door bothers you, lay a towel against the door.

- **Keep it natural.** If you want to wake up shortly after sunrise and the evening lights don't bother you, draw back the heavy curtains before going to bed so the morning sunlight will wake you up naturally. Be sure to check the sunrise schedule for your city.

- **Pack a eye mask.** It's always a good idea to carry an eye mask, even if you don't use one regularly. Once, the contractor I was working for registered me at a hotel that was on the National Register. At bedtime, I discovered there weren't any shades or blinds, just shear curtains. When I called downstairs, the owner said it was not an oversight – she wanted authenticity. I, for one, don't appreciate authenticity if the sun comes up at 5am and I don't have to be up till 7! Eye masks also come filled with scents – lavender and vanilla are said to be relaxing scents.

- **Carry a nightlight.** Do you ever wake up in the night to use the bathroom? Instead of the bright bathroom light, which can wake you up, bring along a nightlight. Even better, *SharperImage©* (www.sharperimage.com) has this fabulous Color Flow™ Light Show nightlight that provides just a mist of colored light or an ever-changing spectrum of color. It helps to show you the way without lighting up the room.

- **Wake up without a jolt.** Part of getting a good night's sleep is waking up without the scare of an unfamiliar alarm clock. Even if you don't need to set the alarm, make sure the previous resident doesn't still have it set for 4 am. To prevent the early morning jolt, consider using the same brand alarm clock at home and on the road. There are plenty of travel alarm clocks in stores, catalogs, and online. Some start at a low volume and then build up slowly; others sound like Big Ben. It's also nice to have an alarm clock that wakes you to your favorite CD music. If you sleep very soundly, pack a battery operated alarm clock, set the room alarm, and ask for a wakeup call (or two) as a backup. If there is no wakeup service available or you think you need a second call, dial 1-900-SUNRISE. For just $0.99 you can arrange your own wakeup call and send yourself a reminder of your to-do list for the day.

- **Get into the light.** Since exposure to sunlight during the day helps to reset your internal clock, try to schedule a midday walk outside. If you wake up earlier than you'd like, get some natural daylight exposure late in the day. No opportunity to get outside in the sunlight? Using a lightbox for an hour or two of bright light exposure in the evening (while you're reading or watching television) may help you to sleep longer in the morning. Exposure to these special lights may also be helpful for those suffering from SAD (Sudden Affective Disorder) or jet lag. Northern Light Technologies, as well as other companies, sells travel light boxes (800-263-0066, www.northernlight-tech.com).

- **Stop the noise.** When checking into a hotel request a quiet room. If you get a blank stare, ask a few questions: is it near an elevator? Ice machine? Facing the interstate? Overlooking the pool? It is easier to switch rooms at registration than after you've settled in. Once you've checked in, put out the "Do not disturb" sign. You may even consider canceling the morning paper delivery. That slap on the floor may be waking you up.

- **Make some noise.** Can't get rid of the noise? Then drown it out with the fan and foam ear plugs (be sure your ears are dry before putting in or you could end up with an ear infection). Strange as it sounds, some travelers drown out the noise by tuning the radio for static between stations. Or bring your own sound machine. *SharperImage*® (www.SharperImage.com) has a lightweight travel CD Radio/Alarm Clock with Sound Soother®. There are 20 sounds (including ocean, babbling brook, and jungle) to relax you into sleep or to wake you gently. I like the soft sound of "rain." It's much like the white noise of the air cleaner machine I use at home. The sleep mode timer can be set for 15, 30, 45, or 60 minutes; it doesn't shut down abruptly but gradually ramps down to silence. And if you can't find your glasses, just tap the button and a pleasant voice will speak the time.

▶ **Downshift Your Body to Sleep.** We all know the benefits of getting children ready for bed with a nightly routine, such as a night snack, brushing their teeth, and reading a story. Our bodies, too, need to be programmed that it is time for sleep.

- **Establish your nightly routine.** Your nightly routine also acts as Zeitgebers to help shift your body down into neutral. Get into your pajamas, have a night snack, brush your teeth, turn the lights down, set the alarm or ask for a wakeup call, put away the heavy work stuff, and opt for some light reading. Begin the routine early; washing your face right before lights out might just wake you up again.

- **Keep to consistent hours.** Whenever possible, keep to a consistent bedtime and wake time. If you're sleep deprived, it's best to go to bed earlier and wake up at your normal time. Sleeping in on your days off may be tempting, but only makes it more difficult to get to sleep at a regular time on business days.

- **Cross time zones without breaking down.** As a general rule, it takes one day for your body to adjust to each time zone you cross. If you are traveling over time zones and the trip is just a few days long, it is may be best to keep your sleep/wake schedule to your home times. If this is impossible due to your work schedule, consider adjusting your body to the time schedule of where you will be traveling to a day in advance – or a *few* days in advance if you are traveling across several time zones. If that's too drastic of a change try splitting the difference. For example, if you're traveling from NY to LA (3 hours earlier) go to bed one and a half hours later for a night or two before you leave so you'll just have another one and a half hours to adjust when you arrive.

- **Beds are for sleeping.** If you can fall asleep easily on a sofa or chair, then find it difficult to fall asleep in bed, you may be associating the bed with everything but sleep. To re-program your association, don't use the bed for business reading or computer work. Watch TV or read in the chair. Work at the desk. Then get into the bed only when you're tired.

▶ **Get Comfortable.** Let's face it, it's difficult to get to sleep if you're uncomfortable. Here are some things to consider before bedtime.

- **Clear your nose.** Nasal congestion and allergies can make sleep uncomfortable. Check with your physician about medications that can help, but be sure they don't have a stimulating effect. If allergies wake you up midmorning (when pollen counts are often the highest) consider taking your usual allergy pill before bedtime.

- **Bring your own pillow and/or pillow case.** Some travelers say they can sleep anywhere if they have their own pillow or just the pillowcase. It's been rumored that George W Bush carries his own feather pillow. Too bulky, you say? To save space, buy a specialty plastic bag that takes the air out so your pillow (or any bulky item) packs more compactly. Several brands and their sources are listed in the *Getting Your Wheels in Gear* chapter. If you forget your own pillow and the ones offered aren't to your liking, call housekeeping to see if they have others – perhaps a feather pillow? I find many hotel pillows uncomfortable – they're too fluffy. So I take along a small camping pillow.

- **Warm feet, cold room.** Adjusting the temperature to about 65 degrees is said to contribute to a good night's sleep. Warm hands and feet also help. Increased blood flow to the hands and feet means the body's core temperature drops, a necessary trigger for sleep. So put on your warm socks!

- **Get out of the rut.** Some hotel mattresses are well-worn, especially on the side where the nightstand and phone are located. Check out your bed and pick a spot with more support and less wear. Consider sleeping on the diagonal. Also check that the sheets are tucked in the best they can be. Getting short-sheeted in the middle of the night can disrupt your sleep.

▶ **Relax.** For many people that's easier said than done, but with practice I believe each of us can be successful. The key is finding the method that works for you. You can either start by relaxing your mind which relaxes your body. Or you can focus on relaxing your body - and your mind will then follow. Here are a few ideas on how to accomplish this:

- **Read a book.** Just don't pick one that will encourage you to stay up until the wee hours of the night.

- **Listen to sweet sounds.** Bring your favorite relaxing music.

- **Practice yoga or meditation.** They help to relax the mind *and* the body. Carol Dickman's Bedtop Yoga is an audiotape with simple poses that you can do on your bed (1-888-YES-YOGA).

- **Take some help along.** There are a variety of CDs and audio relaxation tapes that actually lead you to a state of relaxation. The key is to select one that has a pleasant voice and a machine that doesn't click at the end and wake you back up. Sound machines, not only drown out unwanted noise, but are also very relaxing. Elaine Petrone (www.elainepetrone.com, 800-649-6846) offers a Ball Therapy kit. Using two therapy balls, a video demonstration tape, and an audio tape, this system shows you how to remove excess muscle tension from your body.

- **Take a soak.** Why does a warm bath promote sleep? It may be due to the water's relaxing properties or the fact that it promotes your core body temperature to drop. Both signal the body that it's time to sleep.

- **Can't sleep? Don't just lie there cursing.** If you don't fall asleep within 15 minutes, get out of bed and do some light reading, listen to music, or journal until you get tired. Don't work. While others may be able to read themselves to sleep in bed, insomniacs should keep the association of bed and sleep clear. When you're sleepy, get back into the bed.

- **Don't look at the clock.** Anxiously watching the clock while focusing on how much time you have left to sleep may actually cause insomnia. Set your alarm, then turn the face away from your vision. Put away your watch, too.

- **Have sweet thoughts.** When you say to yourself "I can't sleep. I'll never get to sleep. I'm going to be exhausted tomorrow." Guess what? You won't be able to sleep! Why? It's simple. Those negative, worrying thoughts cause a release of adrenaline which has a stimulating effect. So think relaxing thoughts. Picture yourself in a

79

tub of hot water, floating on a cloud, or at your favorite vacation spot. Other people relax by imagining themselves fishing, deciding what they would do if they won a million dollars, or designing their own dream home.

- **Put your worries down on paper.** Not surprising, the 2000 NSF Poll found that 34% of women and 22% of men said stress affects their sleep. If your thoughts turn to worries when the lights go out, keep a notebook on the nightstand. Before retiring, write down everything you need to do the next day. Also keep a list of your "worries" and jot down some possible solutions. When you wake up worrying, calm yourself down by repeating: "It's OK, I've written it down. There's nothing I can do right now."

- **Connect with your loved ones.** Carry personal stationary and stamps with you. At the end of the day, instead of turning on the TV, write letters to your relatives and friends. Those thoughts will fill your lonely hotel room and you can go to sleep feeling loved. You may even ask your loved one to give you the wakeup call from home.

▶ **Ask for Directions.** If the tips in this chapter don't help you feel more rested, it's time to get some professional help.

- **See the professionals.** Keep a sleep diary to share with your doctor. There may be an underlying causes such as sleep apnea that can be successfully treated or controlled once properly diagnosed. Sleep apnea is a condition whereby the muscles of the throat relax to the point of blocking the windpipe. This will cause chronic, loud snoring coupled with frequent and long pauses in breathing. In addition to promoting excessive daytime sleepiness, sleep apnea can contribute to serious heart problems, high blood pressure, and stroke. Sufferers of sleep apnea are up to seven times more likely to fall asleep at the wheel, three times more likely to be involved in a collision in a five year period, and five times more likely to be involved in multiple crashes. For a sleep apnea questionnaire and other information, check out www.apneanet.org.

- **Sleep aids?** If you think you need a sleep aid, talk to your doctor. Unfortunately, many prescription sleeping pills are addictive or can make you feel groggy in the morning. For that reason, many people seek their local pharmacy for a more "natural" supplement. Regardless of what claims are present or implied, dietary supplements are not regulated by the US Food and Drug Administration (FDA). Under the US Dietary Supplement Health and Education Act of 1994, "dietary supplements" do not need FDA approval, their manufacture is not controlled for quality (as drug manufacturers are), and long term studies of safety are not required. Valerian, a herb supplement, taken at bedtime appears to have minimal side effects, but the US Pharmacopeial Convention which sets standards for drugs, says "the use of valerian for longer than two weeks is not recommended" and suggests people who take it for three months or longer might want to get periodic liver function tests. Another supplement, Melatonin, a synthetic hormone sold as a food supplement, is not recommended. Few studies have been done on melatonin's safety, effectiveness, side effects, interactions with other drugs, and long-term effects. Most researchers agree that the available dosages of this hormone supplement are too high to be safe.

Dr Jo's D.R.E.A.M. Formula

I used to have problems relaxing and getting a good night's sleep so I developed this five step process that guides me into a peaceful sleep every time. Give it a try.

- **Deep breathing** – Have you ever watched a baby sleep? When sleeping babies are placed on their back, their chest expands and deflates dramatically. When you take deep breaths, focus on the same body movement. Your chest and waist should expand, but your shoulders should not rise. Focus on a pattern that increasingly gets deeper and slower. Start with a timing of perhaps three slow counts in and out. It helps to silently count your breaths: "in, 2, 3, out, 2, 3." After that gets comfortable, increase the length to 4 counts.

- **Relaxation** – Once your breathing slows down, begin to relax your body. With each outgoing breath focus on stress and tension leaving your body. Work either from the toes up or from the head down. I find it easier to relax from the top down since I carry most of my stress in my face, neck, and upper back. For example, with your next outgoing breath, focus on releasing and relaxing your forehead. On the next breath, relax your cheeks, then your jaw. Don't rush; it's OK to stay on the same part of the body for several (or more) breaths. Work on down to your neck, shoulders, arms, chest, belly, thighs, calves, and finally down to your toes.

- **Erase negative thoughts from your mind** – As your body begins to relax (even if you're not down to your toes yet), go onto the next step. Release negative and annoying thoughts from your mind by first recognizing these thoughts and then letting them go. Every time a thought (with it's resulting picture) pops into your head, try one of the following imaging techniques: watch it drift off on a white, fluffy cloud; put those thoughts into a box and place it on a shelf; erase it with an old-fashioned chalkboard eraser; or paint over those thoughts with a paint roller and white paint. Don't be surprised if negative, stressful thoughts continue to pop into your mind. Just keep on repeating the image. Or feel free to go back to focusing on the deep breathing or the relaxation.

- **Affirmation** – Thoughts and worries that keep you awake may never completely go away. Keep focusing on letting them go. Then begin to replace them with a positive affirmation such as "relax," "peace," "calm," or "I am sleepy."

- **Mental picture** – Lastly, picture a relaxing thought (such as a beach, mountain scene, a water fountain, a pleasant childhood or vacation memory, or a leaf floating slowly down a fresh water stream). Even if you're still having a problem erasing your negative thought, allow this relaxing thought to override. Other people have shared stories of how they mentally rearrange the furniture in their house or imagine themselves getting ready for a trip. If these ideas sound strange, find something else that's relaxing for you.

Recharge Your Batteries with A PowerNap

Although sleep is the only solution for the sleep-deprived, many people report that a short nap energizes them much like rebooting your computer system when it gets locked up. I have been powernapping since my college days – it gives me the alertness I need for an upcoming meeting or a long car trip. Give it a try!

▶ **Find a Comfortable Place.** Although experienced powernappers can snooze in a busy airport or a noisy hotel lobby, if you've never tried powernapping it'll be important to find a comfortable, quiet space. It could be at your desk or in your car with the seat reclined. If the boss isn't keen on you napping in your office, excuse yourself to the restroom. When you're desperate, you can sit on the toilet and rest your head on your folded arms in your lap.

▶ **Follow Dr Jo's D.R.E.A.M. Formula.** Close your eyes and follow Dr. Jo's D.R.E.A.M. formula. Keep naps to 10-20 minutes (set your watch alarm). Longer naps will pull you into a deeper state of sleep and can have the opposite effect of making you feel drugged and may negatively affect your night sleep. Some people say they fall asleep for just a minute (or even less) and wake up refreshed. One short method is to relax in a chair with a pen in your hand. When you fall asleep and the pen hits the floor, the noise will wake you.

▶ **Stay Safe.** If you're napping at the airport, keep a luggage strap around your leg. If you're on the road pull your car into a safe place, preferably a busy restaurant rather than a rest stop – and lock up. I've had people say "Don't you know how dangerous it is to nap in your car?" My response is always the same, "It's less dangerous or certain than wrapping my car around a power pole on the side of the road." When I'm *that* tired, all I need is a quick powernap to get home safely.

Sweet dreams!

Chapter 4

Fine Tuning Your Engine

In This Chapter:

▶ Common Traveler's Ailments including jet
   lag, motion sickness, & traveler's diarrhea
▶ *Dr Jo's Prescription for Keeping Your
   Energy Up All Day Long*

Being sick at home is no fun, but getting sick on the road
can be a nightmare. While proper maintenance will help to
prevent most breakdowns, if you travel a lot you'll eventually get sick. Here are a few tools to help you survive the
journey.

Common Traveler's Ailments

▶ **Ear Pain.** The air pressure of the cabin can make it difficult to equalize the pressure behind your middle ear causing
pain. What to do?

- **Unstuff your nose**. It's best to avoid flying if you have a
  cold or severe allergies. If you must fly, check with your
  doctor. They will probably recommend an antihistamine
  and/or decongestant medication plus a nasal decongestant spray to be used just before take off and landing.
  Keep in mind that decongestant nasal sprays can be ad-

dictive when used more than a couple of days consecutively. A more natural method is to rub eucalyptus oil on your hands and cup them over your nose to open up your sinuses on takeoffs and landings.

- **Yawn often.** Equalize the pressure in your eustacian tubes by swallowing and yawning. Bring along some chewing gum or a hard candy for take off and landings. Or try this three step process. First, pinch your nostrils shut and take in a breath of air. Without opening your nose or mouth, force air into your nose by gently trying to "blow" your nose. You should hear a pop when you've succeeded.

▶ **Swollen Ankles.** Puffy ankles are caused by lack of circulation from sitting too long in a car, bus, train, or plane. Prolonged sitting also increases our risk of developing deep vein thrombosis (DVT), blood clots that can travel to our lungs and kill us. Here's what to do for swollen ankles:

- **Move around often.** When driving, take a break every two hours. Instead of pulling up to the drive-through, get up and walk around for 10-15 minutes. On a bus, train, or plane (as long as the ride is stable) get up every hour or so and walk around. If that is not possible, do a few exercises in your seat. Roll onto your toes, back onto your heels, and rotate your ankles in both directions.

- **Buy big shoes.** If your feet swell so much that you can't get your shoes back on, buy your travel shoes a half size larger than you need, plus a pair of insoles (available at most drug stores). Go ahead and slip your shoes off. If they are hard to get back on, take out the insoles and your shoe will fit until your feet go back down to normal size.

- **Hold the salt.** High sodium foods like Bloody or Virgin Marys, french fries, pretzels, and peanuts are only going to make the swelling worse. Order a low sodium meal on your flight and carry your own fresh fruit. In addition, since our body is 60% water, it's critical to drink plenty of water. In addition to swollen ankles, being dehydrated will also make you feel sluggish and fatigued.

- **See your doctor.** Deep vein Thrombosis (DVT) is serious. Pregnant women and women taking hormones (birth-control pills or hormone-replacement therapy) appear to be at a greater risk. Doctors may suggest that travelers with an increased risk take aspirin or other blood thinners before flying, or wearing compression stockings. If you're experiencing DVT-like symptoms see your doctor. Be sure to mention that you've been traveling.

▶ **Respiratory Infections.** Airplanes have unhealthy air. The low humidity (typically under 10%) combined with the mostly recycled air makes you more susceptible to getting respiratory infections. If you have a cold, your fellow travelers would appreciate it if you'd keep your germs to yourself and not fly. Here's what you can do to combat the unhealthy air on airplanes:

- **Drink plenty of water.** Because it's easy to get dehydrated, keep a bottle of water with you at all times. So you don't forget, have an outside pocket in your briefcase reserved for your personal water bottle. Grab a bottle on the way out the door, buy one from the snack bar near the gate, or bring your own (empty) bottle and fill it yourself at the water fountain. If you forget, ask the flight attendant upon boarding, they'll often provide you with a glass or bottle even before takeoff.
- **Avoid alcohol and caffeinated beverages.** These only dehydrate you further.
- **Moisturize.** Moist mucous membranes help to fend off colds. So, use a saline nasal spray. Since the low humidity on planes can cause uncomfortably dry eyes, artificial tear drops can help. In addition, remove your contact lenses or have your lens case readily available if you need to remove them.
- **Wash your hands frequently.** Viruses can live for hours on surfaces such as telephones, doorknobs, and on the last hand you shook. So wash your hands thoroughly and frequently, like before removing your contact lenses.

87

Carry antiseptic lotion or wipes with you for the times when soap and water are not available. And keep your hands away from your eyes, nose, and mouth.

- **Ask to be reseated.** If your seatmate is sneezing and coughing, ask to be reseated. It really isn't rude to not want to share his cold. No other seats? Cover your mouth and nose when they sneeze.

- **Stay away from smoking.** Ask to be seated in the non-smoking section in restaurants, take nonsmoking flights (some non-domestic flights still permit smoking), and stay away from smokers in public places. And don't smoke yourself!

- **Try vitamin C, echinacea, and zinc lozenges.** Echinacea may help your body fend off a cold or flu, while Vitamin C and zinc may help to reduce symptoms of a cold. Don't take them on a regular basis. Instead, "shock" your system by taking only upon the symptoms of a cold. Although determined dosages have not been established, try 500-2000 mg of Vitamin C/day when you develop symptoms.

- **Seek medical attention if your symptoms are severe.** Antibiotics won't work on colds and other viruses. But they may be needed if you then get a secondary ear, sinus, or lung infection.

▶ **Motion Sickness.** We experience motion sickness (including nausea and vomiting) when our brain receives conflicting information about our balance and body position. When you experience the initial symptoms such as drowsiness, fatigue and queasiness in your stomach, respond with these suggestions:

- **Move to a stable location.** If you're on a ship or plane, move to the center where it tends to be more stable. Simply closing your eyes and relaxing can be very effective against nausea. On a boat or ship, go up to the top deck and look out at the water to put your eyes and inner ear in sync. If you experience motion sickness frequently, practice relaxation on a regular basis so you'll get a quick response.

- **Move to the front.** In a car, move to the front seat or at least face forward and get some fresh air by opening the window. Look at the horizon and avoid reading. It may also help to close your eyes or stop the car and take a break from moving.

- **Eat lightly, but avoid alcohol.** Pay attention to what you eat – you may find some foods soothing and others may bring on nausea.

- **Try ginger.** Ginger is a traditional Chinese herbal remedy and is available in pills, chewable gingerroot, and candied. Side effects seem to be minimal but it's always wise to still check with your doctor since it has been shown to have some blood-thinning effects. P.S. There isn't enough ginger in gingerale to be effective.

- **Ask your doctor for medication.** There are many medications (both over-the-counter and prescription) that prevent or treat nausea and vomiting. Each have side effects and may cause interactions with other medications. Over-the-counter medications which prevent motion sickness include meclizine (*Bonin*) and dimenhydrinate (*Dramamine*). Prescription meds include *Transderm Scop* (a prescription patch placed behind the ear in advance of symptoms) to prevent motion sickness and promethazine (*Phenergan*) for treating motion sickness.

- **Try a preventive device.** Although not scientifically proven, there are wrist bands that provide electrical stimulation or accupressure. As with every other unscientifically proven device or supplement, it's wise to use common sense and check with your doctor to see if it would harm you. Even if there is no medically proven benefit, it may work through the placebo effect.

- **Grab a motion sickness bag.** When all else fails, be ready.

▶ **Traveler's Diarrhea.** Traveler's diarrhea involving abdominal cramping is very common especially when traveling in developing countries. Nearly all cases are caused by infectious agents such as viruses, bacteria, and protozoa which are spread through fecally-contaminated food and water. There are no vaccines to prevent diarrhea so heed these tips to prevent becoming infected:

- **Log onto www.cdc.gov/travel.** The Center for Disease Control has information specific to the countries on your trip.

- **Drink only safe beverages.** Ask local contacts about the purity of tap water and even some bottled water. Safe beverages include bottled beer, wine, alcohol, carbonated beverages, and coffee and hot tea made from boiled water. If you're unsure, it's best to boil the water for at least a minute, use chemical disinfective agents, or a filtration system found in camping supply stores. Remember to use safe water for brushing your teeth as well.

- **Wash your hands frequently.** And keep them away from your mouth, eyes, and nose.

- **Avoid specific foods.** Where sanitation may be poor, avoid eating raw foods (including seafood, salads, and unpeeled fresh fruit), undercooked food, and unpasterized juice, milk, and milk products such as cheese.

- **Ask your doctor for advice before you leave**. In one study, bismuth subsalicylate (*Pepto Bismol*) was shown to reduce the incidence by about 60 percent when the dosage was taken four times a day. Don't take it if you cannot take asprin (it contains asprin) or have kidney insufficiency, gout, or a history of ulcers. Side effects include nausea and constipation, temporary blackening of tongue or stools, and ringing in the ears. Other doctors recommend *Imodium* or *Lomotil*. These medications can be used for a day or two to slow down the frequency of the diarrhea but doesn't get rid of the infection and may sometimes make it worse by keeping the infection inside. Never use these if you have a fever or blood in your stools. Although each of these medications are available over-the-counter, always check with your doctor before treating yourself.

If you get traveler's diarrhea:

- **Seek medical attention** when the diarrhea lasts more than two days or is accompanied by a high fever, blood, mucous, or worms in your stool.

- **Stay hydrated.** No matter what is causing the diarrhea, it's important to stay hydrated. Make sure the water is safe (use bottled or boiled water). It's easier to drink more when the water is flavored. Rehydration solutions are best since they more closely match the electrolytes in your body. If they're not available, use clear soda, juice, *KoolAid*®, or similar products.

- **Watch what you eat.** Avoid foods that worsen the diarrhea, such as heavy spices, greasy foods, and buffets (since foods are often kept at a perfect temperature for bacteria to grow). Stay away from dairy products during the diarrhea and for several days later since the enzymes that digest the natural sugars in milk are destroyed with diarrhea and may take a few days to rejuvenate. Start with simple foods such as bananas, rice, applesauce, and toast (BRAT diet) or salted crackers.

- **Take an antibiotic with you.** If you're going out of the country for an extended period of time, you may want to get a prescription for antibiotics to treat bacteria and protozoa (giardia and amoeba). Fill the prescriptions at home and carry the antibiotics (in its original prescription container) with you in your carry-on bag. Don't take these as preventative medicine; take it if you have three or more loose stools in an eight hour period. Remember that antibiotics do not work on viruses or parasites.

How to Stay Healthy & Fit on the Road

▶ **Jet Lag.** As we discussed in the *Setting the Snooze Control* chapter, our internal body clock is regulated by circadian rhythms that respond to daily light/dark cycles. When we travel over time zones, these abrupt changes confuse your body clock and cause what is referred to as jet lag. Symptoms of jet lag include fatigue, sleep problems, irritability, queasiness, upset stomach, headache, and grogginess or difficulty concentrating. Jet lag symptoms appear to be more severe (and can last more than a week) when flying east or crossing three or more time zones. To prevent jet lag:

- **Start out well-rested.** Get plenty of sleep the night before the trip and pack early so you're not packing at 2am before a 7am flight.

- **Drink plenty of water.** Drink water before, during, and after the flight (aim for at least 8oz per hour). Since dehydration worsens the jet lag symptoms, carry a bottle with you on board. Don't like the taste of water? Try drinking more fruit juices, decaffeinated coffee or tea (caffeine can dehydrate you further), or sodas without caffeine. Go easy on the alcohol; besides being dehydrating, it will also disturb your sleep pattern.

- **Set your clock to your destination.** Since your circadium rhythm is reset by time cues called zietgebers, it's important to set your watch ahead to the new time zone and start thinking of your destination – especially when traveling east. Adjust your eating and sleeping to the new zone. This includes eating breakfast even when it feels like dinner and forcing yourself to stay awake when you want to sleep. Or adjust it as close as you can – even an hour or two will help. The best evening meal to promote sleepiness is one high in carbohydrates such as fruits, sugars, and starchy foods such as bread, pasta, and rice. You may want to bring a high carbohydrate snack with you if you're flying in the evening.

- **Exercise.** Stretching at your seat or walking around the cabin help to ease swelling and muscle cramps and decrease your risk of DVT. Exercise when you arrive may also allow your body to reset your circadian rhythms.

- **Sleep on the "red eye."** If you're taking the "red eye" flight that travels through the night, try to get some sleep even if you're not yet tired. It helps to use ear plugs, eye mask, and neck pillow (the inflatable ones take up less room) and to ask for a window seat so no one will step over you. Dress in comfortable clothing and don't stay up to watch the movie.

- **Stay up if it's daytime at your destination.** If it's daytime at your destination, even if you feel like sleeping, force yourself to stay awake by reading a mystery novel, playing a game, or talking to your neighbors. To keep alert, eat a high protein/low carbohydrate meal like meat, vegetables, and only small amounts of carbohydrates like bread, rice, and noodles. Caffeine (coffee, tea, and caffeinated sodas) may also help to keep you awake. But don't overdo the caffeine if you'll be needing to fall asleep soon.

- **Join the Airline Club Rooms.** Upon arriving on a "red eye" flight, you'll feel more refreshed if you can shower and change into your business clothes.

- **If you're tired, take a short nap.** If you arrive in their morning (your middle of the night) you may feel like sleeping all day, but then you'll be on the wrong schedule. You can stay up all day and get to bed early that night but sleeplessness can be very disorienting and dangerous. Instead, take just a short nap of no more than three hours. Then take a shower, go for a walk, and get something to eat. You'll feel a bit more refreshed but still ready to go to bed at your new bedtime.

- **Get some sun.** Spend half an hour or so outside in the daylight walking around as soon as you arrive (or the next morning if you're arriving at night). For east to west travelers, take a walk in the late afternoon. Can't get outside? Spend time next to windows. Indoor lights are not bright enough to make a difference; if jet lag is a frequent problem, you may want to invest in a traveler's size lightbox (www.northernlights-tech.com).

How to Stay Healthy & Fit on the Road

- **Pace yourself.** If your schedule permits, allow yourself some time to rest and relax before touring or conducting business. Save the important activities for when you have the most energy – in the mornings after flying west and in the evening after flying east.

- **Talk to your doctor about medications.** Some travelers take sleeping pills during the flight to induce sleep. Unfortunately, medications can cause disorientation the next morning (and on the flight if there is an emergency).

- **Be cautious of "natural" remedies.** There are several so-called "natural remedies" for jet lag found in stores. As discussed in the last chapter, these "dietary supplements" are not regulated by the Food and Drug Administration (FDA). So although they may have claims, these do not have to be backed by research for proof of effectiveness or long-term safety. Keep in mind that even if these so-called "jet lag" therapies seems to work, the effect may simply be a placebo effect. The herb Valerian appears to be safe for short-term use in inducing a relaxed state. While there are anecdotal reports of effectiveness, no studies have yet demonstrated that melatonin (a hormone) relieves jet lag in a measurable way compared to placebo (or sugar pill) treatment alone. Light resets the body's rhythms or biological clock in a more powerful way than melatonin – and light offers no side effects or long term safety issues.

- **Naturally induce sleep.** Lowering the body temperature seems to help make you sleepy, so take a warm bath (one hour before bedtime) and wear socks in bed if your feet get cold.

▶ **Altitude Sickness**. If you'll be climbing mountains, remember that air pressure falls as you climb above sea level. When you climb over 8000 feet, less oxygen is available to your tissues – commonly referred to as "thin air." This causes a normal adaptation process involving more frequent breathing, increased heart rate and pulse, dryness of skin and mucous membranes, and minor headache. When the ascension is too rapid, some people experience Acute Mountain Sickness (AMS) resulting in shortness of breath and/or cough, headache, chest discomfort, nausea, vomiting, fatigue and sleeplessness, disorientation and loss of coordination. These symptoms usually develop within 36 hours at that elevation. In severe cases which involve swelling of the brain and/or fluid in the lungs, sufferers are unable to walk a straight line, become disoriented, and can lapse into a coma and die. To prevent AMS:

- **Drink plenty of fluids**
- **Avoid alcohol and tobacco**
- **Get in shape prior to your trip**
- **Climb slowly.** Start your trip below 10,000 feet and ascend no more than 1000 feet per day. If you climb more than 1000 feet in a day, sleep at a lower altitude. Take a day of rest every 3000 feet climbed.
- **Ask your doctor about prevention therapy** such as *Diamox* – a diuretic which is prescribed before and during your climb. It cannot be taken by persons allergic to sulfa drugs.

Dr Jo's Prescription for
Keeping Your Energy Up All Day Long

Probably one of the most common physical complaints that travelers have is that of being tired. You too? Well, read on.

For my masters degree in Human Nutrition from Virginia Polytechnic Institute, I conducted research on "Ideopathic Migraines and Impaired Glucose Tolerance." Along with an otolaryngologist, we looked at 125 people who had migraines for no apparent physiological reason. In the complete physical we noticed that nearly all had some form of impaired glucose responses including diabetes or hypoglycemia (low blood sugar).

When placed on a balanced nutritional program (described later), these patients improved their glucose and insulin responses and noted a significant decrease in the number and severity of their migraines. In addition, I heard so many people remark at how much more energy they had.

I was so convinced, that I begin eating like my study participants. And I still follow this plan – more than 20 years later. I lost the ten pounds that I was always struggling with and I've kept my weight stable for these twenty plus years. If you want more energy, the following pages provide some tips to help you too.

▶ **Treat Yourself Right.**
- **Understand your own personal energy cycle** – for most people energy levels peak around noon and then goes through a slump in mid-afternoon. Instead of fighting your personal low, work around it by getting critical tasks done when you feel your best and doing more routine tasks when you're in a slump.
- **Take care of your needs.** Are you overworked? Do you try to keep everyone happy at the expense of your own needs? Do you have any hobbies or allow yourself to

have fun every once in a while, or is your life work, work, work? Do you spend time with friends you enjoy? When we spend too much time giving to others and not to ourselves, it eventually drains us of our energy. We'll discuss this in greater detail in chapter eight, *Staying Balanced*.

- **Make sleep a priority.** Are you getting enough sleep? If you wake up refreshed without an alarm clock you're probably getting enough. If you don't feel refreshed, try getting to bed a half-hour earlier each night. Having a hard time getting to sleep? Follow the tips in the *Setting the Snooze Control* chapter.

- **Learn to powernap.** Even when you can't get in a full night's sleep, a short powernap midday can help make you feel energized.

- **Manage your stress.** Don't take on more than you can handle and don't procrastinate. Avoid the panic mode as much as possible. Although the release of adrenaline can create a temporary "high," it comes at a price. When things settle down, like at the end of the day or work week, we find ourselves completely fatigued. Read the *Putting the Brakes on Stress* chapter. There you'll learn tips on how to respond differently to stressful situations so you can prevent this rebound reaction.

- **Get outside.** Sometime during each day breathe in fresh air, feel the sun, and listen to the birds. And leave your cell phone behind. Even a few minutes outside will help you to slow down your pace!

- **Get regular exercise.** Exercise is proven to reduce stress and make you feel more in control. If you're not already exercising on a regular basis, find an activity that works for you. Some like to pound the pavement, while others find slow laps in the pool to be more relaxing. According to research, exercise can be just as effective as medication in improving your mood and giving you more energy – and it's a great deal healthier.

▶ **Follow a Healthy Eating Pattern.** This is the dietary program we gave to our study participants:

- **Keep to a regular eating schedule.** Busy people and travelers tend to allow people and events to get in the way of a regular schedule. Make eating a priority.

- **Eat breakfast** even if you don't feel like it. Eat within the first hour (or preferably the first 30 minutes) of waking. If you have breakfast planned with others later, eat something small beforehand. Try a banana, Dr Jo's "Breakfast in a cup," or nibble on a bagel.

- **Eat every three hours.** Some of us, whether we have true hypoglycemia or are just overly sensitive to the normal swings in our blood sugar, feel better when we eat every three hours. I gave the participants a plan that included three small meals plus three snacks. For inactive people, it was just a small 100-150 calorie snack (see *Fueling the Engine* chapter) such as six crackers with an ounce of cheese, a cup of sugar-free yogurt, glass of skim or lowfat milk, sugar-free hot cocoa, or a *Glucerna*® or *Ensure*® bar. More active people were given larger 200-300 calorie snacks like a handful of nuts or a half of a bagel.

- **Include protein at every meal.** Breakfast may include a glass of milk (or yogurt) and egg (or egg substitutes). At lunch and dinner, include a small portion (about the size of a deck of cards) of beef, chicken, fish, cheese, or soy protein about the size of a deck of cards. Remember to enjoy the low fat versions for health.

- **Limit the number of carbohydrates you have at each meal.** Carbohydrates are not bad for you; they provide much needed energy in a healthy way. When we eat carbohydrates, our blood sugar rises. In response, the pancreas produces insulin which escorts the carbohydrates from the blood stream into our body's cells.

However, when we eat too much carbohydrates at a time, some of us may overproduce the insulin - and our blood sugar drops extremely low. Although true hypoglycemia (under 50 mg/dl) is rare, some of us may feel the "drops" when if it falls too fast or to a level such as 60 or 70 mg/dl. Symptoms include: sleepiness, confusion, headaches, and inability to concentrate. If that sounds like you, simply limit the number of carbohydrates that you have at a time. If you're inactive, have no more than three servings at each meal and one or two at a snack. Active people can handle more; keep to no more than five servings at each meal and two or three at a snack.

That may sound like a lot, but a typical meal at a Mexican restaurant (chips, rice, beans, and tortillas) could easily provide ten servings. One serving is: a small piece of fruit or ½ cup canned fruit, ½ cup juice or soda, one slice bread, ½ english muffin, ¼ large deli bagel, ¾ c cereal, ½ cup noodles or rice, ½ cup of starchy vegetables (potatoes, corn, peas, beans), three cups of popcorn, 10 chips, one small cookie, six crackers, four pieces of hard candy, or a thin slice of cake.

- **Keep the concentrated amounts of sugar to 1-2 servings a day.** While concentrated forms of simple sugar (such as soda, cookies, candy), can raise and then drop your sugar, there's no physiological reason to cut out all sugar. Even diabetics are no longer being told to cut out all sugar – sugar isn't as bad as we once thought. Just don't consume it alone on an empty stomach and don't eat all your allotted carbohydrates in the form of simple sugars. Try to avoid these simple sugars for snacks, and only include a small amount in your meal. I found out years ago, that denying myself sugar only makes the urge stronger.
- **Avoid alcohol.** Alcohol can cause low blood sugar.
- **Limit caffeine.** Cut back completely if you think your energy drop might be due to oversensitive blood sugar fluctuations. If your lows are due to not getting a good night's sleep, avoid caffeine completely or drink only a cup or two in the morning – and then none for the rest of the day.

99

▶ **Check With Your Healthcare Team.** If the previous mentioned suggestions aren't working, check with your doctor.

- **Describe your symptoms.** Keep a journal about your day and how you feel. When did you first notice the change? Do you feel sleepy or physically weak? Does your energy wax and wane throughout the day or is it constantly at a low level? Do you have good days and bad days?

- **Get tested.** Many conditions and diseases can totally zap your energy including depression, low testosterone levels, walking pneumonia, sleep apnea, restless leg syndrome, onset of diabetes, heart or lung problems, anemia, thyroid problems, cancer or hormonal changes due to menopause. Discuss having a glucose tolerance test to check your blood sugar since, as we mentioned, people with diabetes (high blood sugar) as well as hypoglycemia (low blood sugar) can feel wasted.

- **Ask about medications you take.** Drugs to control anxiety and high blood pressure, as well as antihistamines, can drain your energy.

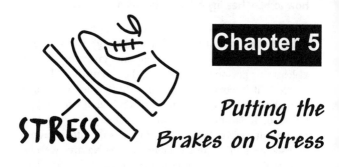

Chapter 5

Putting the Brakes on Stress

In This Chapter:
▶ Do a Pre-Trip Inspection
▶ Heed the Warning Lights - including
  Dr Jo's Quick Tips to Stop Overheating
▶ Avoid the Bumps in the Road
▶ Make the Ride Enjoyable

Most of us run on "automatic" in that our daily actions and reactions are somewhat predictable. We take our shower on automatic, get dressed by putting the same leg into our pants first each and every time, and somehow get home safely even though we don't even remember the drive. So, in many ways, running on automatic makes our life easier.

But running on "automatic" is not healthy if your usual actions and reactions are stressing you out. While there will always be flight delays, road construction, overbearing people, and more work than there is time, these situations, by themselves, don't cause the stress. Don't believe me? The next time you're in a situation that you define as stressful, look around. Chances are, you'll see people that appear perfectly calm. Surely, you've had the opportunity to comment (to another person who heard exactly what you heard or who

101

is stuck in the same situation) something like, "Can you believe that? Isn't it just awful?" Although I can always find someone to commiserate with me, invariably there's at least one person that says "No, that's not what I heard" or "Nah, it'll work out just fine." That's when you begin to realize that situations by themselves don't make you stressed. It is our perceptions of these situations that create our stress. While we can't change other people and we certainly can't change Mother Nature, we *can* change the way we look at things so we have a healthier response to the situation. This chapter includes four steps to help you reprogram your "automatic" transmission.

Dr Jo's Serenity Prayer for Travelers:
God, grant me the wisdom to plan well for things I can control; to retain patience, perspective, and a backup plan when things I can't control go awry; and the ability to laugh when nothing else works.

Do a Pre-Trip Inspection

None of us look forward to our car breaking down on a long trip. So chances are, before a long road trip, you check the tire pressure, the fluid levels, and maybe even take the car in for a tune-up. If you're feeling the pressures of stress, it's time to do a pre-trip inspection of your life as well.

▶ **Remember Why You Work.** It's been said that no one sits on their deathbed wishing they had spent more time at work. On the contrary, most people wish they had spent more time with loved ones. While your job can be satisfying, do you want it to become your whole life?

- **Ask yourself what your priorities are.** Chances are your friends and family will top the list and not your job. Since life is so short, keep faithful to your priorities by investing the necessary time and attention. Or at least put at much effort into your personal life as you do your business life.

- **Spend less than you make.** If you continue to spend more than you make, you'll always need to work harder and harder. Instead, set up a budget that will get your finances under control. Get in the habit of paying your savings account first and buying less stuff. Limit yourself to one or two business and personal credit cards (cancel the rest) and always pay more than the minimum amount to avoid paying excessive credit card interest. If you have a spending problem, get some professional help.

▶ **Set Your Limits.** Do you ever complain about being overworked? Most of us have. It's easy to blame everyone else, but remember that it takes two to tango. Although we can't control what other people do or don't do, ask yourself what your role is in the situation.

- **Just say no.** Have you sold your soul by allowing others to put too much pressure on you? If so, maybe it's time to establish some rules. Ask around, chances are some of your peers have already done so. Set guidelines about how much you're willing to travel, additional time you'll need to makeup for the time away, and how much work you'll take home with you. If you can't say no, tell them what you're willing to do. For example, instead of saying that you will not travel on weekends, tell them that you're willing to take the first flight out on Monday or organize a conference call. If you're always at your boss's beck and call 24/7, he or she will continue to expect it. P.S. It also helps to pick compassionate employers in the first place.

- **Take some responsibility.** I still remember the noticeably pregnant woman who kept saying yes to overtime, then complaining, "Why don't they call someone else? Can't they see I'm tired?" Think about it, if you were the manager and someone had called in sick and you needed a replacement fast, who would you call first? Chances are you wouldn't spend the time calling people who always say no. You'd call the people who frequently

103

agree to work overtime, right? So instead of complaining (to everyone but the people who make the decisions), it's time to take some responsibility for the situation you're in.

- **Learn to delegate**. Do you ever fall into the trap of trying to do everything? Me too! You've probably found out that when you take on too much, some of the important things fall through the cracks. Don't put so much pressure on yourself when others are capable (with a little training, perhaps) of handling these tasks. Now is the time to empower your staff and family members to handle more of the routine tasks and decisions. If you don't have an assistant, consider using a concierge service to run errands for you while you're out of town or calling a temporary service agency for help at your destination. No money? Call your local high school or college. They may offer an intern program and have volunteers available. Or use the kids down the street for a few bucks an hour to do some routine tasks.

- **Stay away from negative people**. Like a pebble thrown into a still pond, the ripples of negativism can be far-reaching. So, as much as possible, minimize the time you spend with people that drag you down.

▶ **Simplify.** Several years ago, I was leading a full-day stress management program to an audience of about 200 in Montreal. Just before the afternoon session was to begin, a beautiful woman with short hair rushed up to me and began to thank me profusely. She said "You probably don't remember, but this morning my hair was past my waist. When you talked about making time by eliminating low priority tasks, I knew what had to be done. Everyday I spent nearly an hour washing, drying, and styling my hair. So I got it cut over the lunch break and I love it!"

Sounds drastic, but she went on to say that although she once enjoyed having long hair, it had become a pain in the neck – literally! Now she was excited that she had created time to get back into an exercise routine. What can you do to simplify your life so you'll have time for your top priorities?

- **Simplify your personal care.** Take a look at the time you spend on personal care. As in the aforementioned case, a wash and wear haircut can save much in time. Some people exercise first thing in the morning so they won't need a second shower in the day. I keep my nails short and unpolished so I don't have to worry about chipped polish or broken nails.

- **Simplify the packing.** Have you ever, on the evening before a trip, frantically started a load of clothes because you didn't have any clean underwear? Frequent travelers should own a month's worth of underwear. Drop your business suits off at the dry cleaner just as soon as you return from a trip so it's ready for your next. My husband owns a dozen black pants and two dozen white shirts so he never runs out of these basics. While I like a bit more color, I only buy wrinkle-resistant suits. I haven't ironed in years!

- **Simply your work.** Cut back to just one business and one personal credit card that offers mileage or other benefits. Keeping the business expenses separate simplifies your expense reports. Buy your stamps by mail – don't ever wait in line! Purchase your office supplies and airline tickets on-line.

- **Throw it out!** Clutter creates stress. Isn't it time to do a Spring cleaning? If you think you don't have time to clean, remember how much time you waste looking for things. Maybe you need to call a professional organizer.

- **Simplify your responses.** Chances are you're already using a signature for your email so you don't have to keep typing in your name and contact info. Are you also taking advantage of email auto-responders and using templates for frequently used forms including quotes, invoices, and reports? If you're responding to an email and it just requires a quick response, put it in the subject box followed by <eom> (end of message) so the recipient doesn't even have to open the mail. If

105

you frequently type the same word, phrase, or paragraph, download Robotype, a free utility that lets you quickly insert your "boilerplace" text in any program by using an abbreviation (www.zdnet.com/downloads/stories/info/0,,000OHO,.html).

▶ **Organize**

- **Maintain just one calendar.** Life can be hectic so keep just one calendar to track both your business and personal life. While some people are still using the old-fashioned tickler files or a stack of index cards to remember everything, chances are you're using a paper organizer, computer program, or PDA (personal digital assistant) such as Palm or Handspring. If your system is not working for you, it's time to make a change. More and more business travelers are using PDAs because they're portable, easily accessible, and maintain thousands of contact information records. Use your organizer to keep toll-free numbers for all airlines, rental cars, and hotel chains as well as running lists of things you need to do.

- **Set alarms.** Program your PDA or computer alarm to remind you to pack your itinerary, print out maps, make a phone call, and to pack files you need. Use the alarm in your personal life to program in birthdays, anniversaries, and other special occasions. If you ever get lost in an activity (like I do) set an alarm to keep you on schedule.

- **Have a place for everything.** Life is easier when we can find what we need. Create files of frequently traveled cities to include city maps, where the taxis are located at the airport, and good running courses. Going to a convention? Don't forget to bring your return address stamper so you don't have to keep filling out the same information. Have you ever left items in a hotel room after checkout or found yourself panicking to check out on time? Make a rule to always put your things in the same place so you don't need to check every crevice of the room to make sure you have everything. Never put anything on the back of the bathroom door – it's sure to be forgotten. And get into the habit of keeping your business expense receipts in the same place so you don't lose any - pick a specific pocket in your briefcase.

- **Streamline the process.** Don't let traveling become a burden. If you haven't yet gotten your packing down to a science, refer to the tips in the next chapter, *Getting Your Wheels in Gear*. Frequent travelers should always keep their luggage somewhat permanently packed and the briefcase regularly stocked with all the essentials. Instead of schlepping stuff to your next out of town meeting, think about what you can ship ahead.

▶ **Keep Up the Routine Maintenance.** Each of these activities have been proven to decrease your stress level:

- **Get enough sleep.** I'm sure you can recall dozens of times when you didn't have enough sleep and you overreacted to a situation. Enough said!
- **Exercise on a regular basis.** Exercise relieves stress, makes you feel in control, and is a good time to brainstorm new approaches, plan your day, or just "zone out."
- **Eat right.** Although our body is better at running off fumes than our car, we'll stay more balanced if we take care of ourselves and take in the fuel that we need.
- **Give yourself some solitude every day.** Use this time for prayer, meditation, inspirational reading, or planning your day. Or just daydream. Some people keep a gratitude log of the things for which they are grateful, funny things that have happened, "angels" they met on the road, and fond memories of the past.
- **Talk it out.** At the end of a stressful day, share it with a listening ear. No one wants to hear about it, you say? Talk to your dog – they always seem to understand. If you're really mad, yell at the mirror – it's hard to keep a straight face for too long. Or take a shower to unload your worries and wash them down the drain. I keep a journal to do my emotional dumping – an unedited emo-

tional catharsis of what I'm feeling. While I have an actual book, most of my journaling is done on a scratch pad and then trashed or written on the computer and never saved. If you need to discuss an issue with another person, it's important to get the anger out first, so the message comes across without all the emotion.

- **Give back to others.** Volunteering can also be surprisingly rewarding. Help out at the church, for your kid's activities, or at the soup kitchen. On a smaller scale, collect all the free things from hotels and conventions and donate them to the shelter in your hometown. You can help even on the road. When you see frazzled travelers – kids screaming, tired older person, someone lost – extend your hand and help. Doesn't that feel good?

- **Express your soul.** There are many activities that rejuvenate our spirits. Consider taking up writing, painting, singing, dancing, or other creative hobby that you can take with you on the road.

- **Foster friendships.** Social interaction is healthy. People who have frequent interactions with friends, colleagues, and even strangers tend to live longer, stay healthier, and get fewer colds. Yet, it's easy for travelers to isolate themselves. Make an effort to strike up a conversation with the person next to you on the plane, in line, or in the elevator. You never know, this person may become a good friend, a business client, or just provide a few laughs and interesting conversation for the road. It's easy to make friends when you join a national club such as the Rotary, the Lion's Club, or the Executive Women's Golf Association. Visiting other local affiliates when you travel can help to create nationwide (or international) bonds, gives you an insider's look at various communities, and can open doors within your business.

- **Have a peaceful transition.** Has this ever happened to you? You're dying to get home, but when you open the door and everyone gathers around you and talks at the same time, you feel like screaming. Because it's easy to become overly tired on a trip, plan for some peaceful transition time before catching up with family and friends or returning to the office. Transition time could be as simple as retiring to the bathroom for a bit of an escape or taking a 15 minute nap. Some people sit in the car for a few minutes or take a brief walk in the park along the way. Find something that works for you.

- **Take some time off.** Traveling too much? Then take a half day off and spend it taking care of things around the house, or just on yourself. I like to pamper myself with a nap on weekends. Who says hotels are just for when you're out of town? Consider spending a night in a local hotel when they have specials so you can get away from the phone and reminders of what needs to be done. Order room service, watch a movie or read, and relax.

- **Treat yourself right.** Before each trip ask yourself what you need most – to catchup on work or some relaxation. Then pack and plan accordingly.

Heed the Warning Lights

It's easy to fall into the same old cycle of: "When in question, when in doubt, run in circles, scream and shout." But excessive worrying and fretting will never get you anywhere. It just takes valuable time away from enjoying life and keeps you from the task at hand. Instead, remember:

▶ **You Can't Control Other People.** Have you ever tried to get your loved one to change a habit that you found annoying? Were you successful? I didn't think so. It's hard enough to convince people who *like* you to change, don't even waste your time trying to change other people.

- **Taking it out on others doesn't work.** Personnel at airlines, car rental companies, and restaurants are disinclined to help irate, rude travelers and most times, the attending personnel have nothing to do with the situation at hand. If you are patient and perhaps offer a smile, doors may open where none existed.

- **Focus on yourself.** The only things you truly *can* control are your own attitude, thoughts, and behaviors. Leave behind your need for perfection, your need to control other people, and do what *you* need to do.

▶ **Don't Blow A Fuse.** If you travel enough, you'll have the opportunity to see people lose control. Sure, some situations may be justified, but doesn't that person look foolish? Vow to yourself to never let that happen to you. These tips provide some "tools" for staying calm:

Dr Jo's Quick Tips to Stop Overheating:

Take a deep breath before you regret. We tend to hold our breath when we're upset. Since our cells need a constant supply of oxygen, it's no wonder we can't think clearly! Concentrate on breathing in through your nose, out through your mouth. Remember you should feel your belly come out; your shoulders shouldn't move.

Count to 10 slowly. Have you ever regretted those words you hastily spoke? In most cases, there's no need to respond right away. Count to 10 before you speak.

Relax. Drop those shoulders and relax your facial muscles – you'll be able to think more clearly about the best course of action. See the *Setting the Snooze Control* chapter for more tips on how to relax.

Sing to yourself. An easy way to calm down is to find yourself a coping theme song. Try: "Don't Worry, be happy," "I feel good", "My Favorite Things", "R.E.S.P.E.C.T.", or "Take this job and shove it."

Take a hike. Before you say or do something that you will regret, take a short walk – to the lobby, outside, or just to the water fountain.

Go to your "happy place." Conjure up a relaxing picture in your mind – a childhood memory, the beach, mountain top, or a tropical island. It'll help you relax and change your perspective.

Think about your options. Real quick, think of not one but 10 things you can do in this situation. Some will be outrageous, but at least one will work.

Dr Jo's Quick Tips to Stop Overheating Fuses (cont.):

Change the scenery. When you and another have reached an impasse, take the discussion to another room, downstairs to the lobby, to the coffee shop, or on a hiking trail. It's amazing how a simple change of scenery can change your (and their) outlook.

Laugh more. Don't take everything so seriously! Joanna Slan, author of *Using Stories and Humor: Grab Your Audience*, once told me "I use traveling as a way to flex my humor muscle. When they ask me at the check-in counter, 'Is this the only bag you have?' I'll say 'This and the ones under my eyes.' They always laugh."

Don't take it personal. Remember that just like you, other people have bad days. Keep that in mind when people offer negative comments or seem to overreact. It's probably not about you at all.

"Cartoonize." A friend of mine worked at a customer service center where he only received calls from angry customers. His blood pressure was so high his doctor told him to quit his job. Instead, when people called, he began to imagine what they were saying in a cartoon format in his head. He no longer got upset. In fact, he found it a bit entertaining, he remembered every detail, and his blood pressure came down.

Take a scream break. Take a walk outside and get it off your chest. If you don't want to make a scene, go to your room and scream into your pillow.

Pull out your victory log. Keep a victory log of the positive praise you've received, an accomplishment you have achieved, and the sale you made. When you're feeling down, take a moment to review the log. See it's not all that bad!

Balance both halves of your brain. If you're feeling time-stressed, do some right brain activities – artwork, singing, dancing. If you're feeling down and depressed, switch to some left brain activities such as number crunching or organizing.

Avoid the Bumps Along the Way

Civil engineers had a great idea when they designed those wakeup bumps on the right side of the road. They can be a lifesaver when you're drifting off the road, but would you ride them for miles, just for the fun of it? Of course not. So when you're out on the road, try to avoid your frequent "bumps" – the things that frustrate you – as much as possible. Since you don't always have complete control over things, ask yourself what you most frequently complain about and come up with a backup plan and/or coping technique for each of these frustrations. Here are a few ideas for some of the bumps we travelers experience:

▶**Traveling is Exhausting:**

- **Map your trip before you leave.** Use the internet (Chapter 9 has some web sites) or get directions from clients before heading out of town. And allow yourself plenty of time to get where you need to go. It's always a good idea to keep a pocket road atlas with you at all times. This is helpful when you've forgotten to map your trip, you need to see the whole city at a glance, or if you need to plan alternate routes because of construction or traffic (www.fhwa.dot.gov has information on traffic and road closures).

- **Make the drive to and from the airport less stressful.** Avoid rush-hour flights that make the commute to and from the airport stressful. Take a limo or taxi to the airport and back; depending on length of trip and cost of parking, it may even be less expensive than driving! Or have a friend or family member drop you off and pick you up at the gate. Traveling is more fun and it's easier to unwind if you know someone will be picking you up.

- **Park in the same area of the same parking lot every time.** That way it's easier to find your car. Not possible? Then, as soon as you find a parking spot (and before you unload), write down the exact location on the back of the parking ticket. Then place your parking

112

ticket in your carry-on bag, purse, or briefcase in the same place everytime. DO NOT place your keys in a bag that will get checked on.

- **Smile.** Smile at the person seated next to you. Because smiles are contagious, there's a good chance that they will smile back. And you know what? You'll feel better! Another reason to smile, is that the person next to you could be the person you're flying in to see.

- **Or don't smile.** Don't want to be bothered? Slip on your headphones when your airline neighbor gets too chatty. Or come up with a line to shut them up. For example, when they ask you what you do, answer: "not much lately, I just got released from prison." Too drastic? Okay, come up with your own line.

- **Dress comfortably.** Even if you're leaving for the airport straight from the office, wear comfortable clothes. We'll talk more about this in the *Getting Your Wheels in Gear* chapter.

- **Practice safe eating.** Don't you just hate it when you stain your clothes even before you arrive at your destination? Leave a stirrer or spoon in your hot beverage. It minimizes the liquid from sloshing around on rough flights. Open food packets like cream and salad dressing away from you and towards the back of the seat in front of you. That way, *you* won't get splattered.

- **Join the Airline Club rooms.** Even if you don't want to buy a membership, consider asking for a day pass. This is great when you have a very long layover. When you take a "red eye" flight, you can shower and change into your business clothes.

- **Get comfortable.** Practice exercises (see *Getting Your Body in Shape* chapter) you can do in your seat to reduce swelling and pain from cramped muscles and reduced circulation. Roll up a blanket to put in the small of your back for lumbar support.

- **Learn how to powernap.** A quick 10-15 minute powernap is a great way to recharge your batteries. Don't know how to do it? Go back to the *Setting the Snooze* chapter.

- **Make the drive comfortable.** If I have more than an hour of driving, I bring along a book-on-tape. This is a great way to have an attitude adjustment. There have been times that I'm so caught up in my book that I rejoice when I get into traffic. "Yes! More time to listen to the story."

- **Allow extra time.** Give yourself a break by allowing plenty of time. Don't book too many meetings back to back and allow extra time for unexpected delays, cancelled flights, or other mishaps.

- **Do it in advance.** Order the iron and ironing board right away even if you won't be using it until the morning. Pre-order breakfast the night before by calling room service. Ask for it to be delivered 5 minutes after your wakeup call. This also provides insurance that if you doze back after the wakeup call, you'll have a second chance for a wakeup.

- **Make it easy on yourself.** Don't use anything but luggage on wheels. Book a hotel in close proximity of where you will be working (you can do a search on-line to find hotels within a certain mile radius of where you're working). You may have to drive a bit more after landing, but the next morning's drive will be less rushed. Although there are certainly advantages to staying at a conference's host hotel, consider staying somewhere else when you need extra down time. Use the concierge to request a great room (call before arrival), line up a massage, skilled limo driver, preferred restaurant, childcare, or takeout food. Don't forget to tip well.

- **Leave your luggage.** If you need to leave one city, go to another, and then return to the first, consider leaving some of your luggage with the concierge. Or if you're always returning back to the same hotel, ask the hotel to store some things until your next return. If you're going to work, but need to return to the hotel to take the shuttle to the airport, leave your bag at the hotel – don't schlep it with you.

- **Select a hotel that has a fine restaurant.** This allows you the convenience of entertaining clients downstairs and then just taking the elevator back to your room. You'll save you time; perhaps even enough to squeeze in a work out.

- **Make it easy to get around.** Instead of stressing over car rentals, ask about complimentary airport and/or hotel shuttles. A cab or other form of public transportation can also be convenient when you are just going to one place on your trip. When you have numerous appointments in diverse locations in one day, consider hiring a limousine rather than a cab. It's easier to have the car waiting for you outside the door rather than having to hail another cab – and surprisingly, a fixed daily limo is often less expensive than numerous cabs.

▶**Uncomfortable Flying Coach?** Can they make the seats any smaller? Here are some survival tips:

- **Get to the airport early.** If you are a frequent flyer, an early check-in makes the difference in getting upgrades to business or first class. The contacts you make in first class are often invaluable to your business. If you're on your return trip home, you may be able to get on an earlier flight.

- **Even if you're not an elite flyer, you can often get upgraded.** When booking with Biztravel.com, be sure to request an upgrade which will be sent on the appropriate date. (You can check in advance which flights have available first-class seats and what the rules are). If there are seats, most airlines will confirm an upgrade for elite travelers hours or days before the flight. Even if you're just regular status, you may be eligible for upgrades. For example, if you're traveling last minute and had to pay full-price for an economy seat, American Airlines will confirm upgrades for regular status flyers.

- **Time your travel.** It's difficult to get upgrades at the beginning or the end of the day or week. Midweek and midday travel is the most likely.
- **Join the club.** Frequent Business Travelers Club (www.fbtc.com) and International Airline Passengers Association (www.iapa.com) negotiate member upgrades with major airlines and other travel companies.

How to Get the Best Seat on the Plane:

Book early. Preferably at least three weeks in advance for the best prices – and best seats.

Call for seat assignments. If seat assignments are not available when you make your reservation, ask when they will be. Don't wait until gate check-in time or you may be stuck in the dreaded middle seat.

Take advantage of elite status in your frequent flier program. You are more likely to get free upgrades to first class or they'll keep the seat next to you vacant if at all possible. The quickest way to get upgrade coupons and elite status is to limit your travel to as few hotel and airline choices as possible.

Make sure your seat reclines. Non-reclining seats are very uncomfortable. When purchasing online or picking up your e-tickets, take a look at the airline seating chart. Rows in the exit aisle and in front of the exit row do not recline. Neither does the last row in the plane.

Consider the advantages of window/aisle seats. Aisle seats are good for extra legroom while window seats are better for napping.

Consider the advantages of front/back of the plane. The plane often loads from the back; so those seats offer the prime overhead bins. On the other hand, since the front generally deplanes first, these seats are preferred when you have a tight connection.

How to Get the Best Seat on the Plane (cont.):

Get the seats with more legroom. Bulkhead seats (the first seats in the main section) offer more space than most other seats. You get more foot room and there's no seatback in your face. On the downside, there's often no space in front of you to stow your briefcase and you may have to share your space with families with small children. Emergency aisles also offer more legroom but you must be able to open the emergency door if needed. Those seats in the middle of the emergency aisle do not recline. These seats are not given out until check-in time, so get there early.

Consider left and right sides. If you're flying coach you don't have much elbowroom. If you plan on writing, consider the left aisle seat if you are right-handed or the right aisle seat if you're left-handed. While you can still get bumped from the aisle, you won't have to continually tuck your elbow in to avoid hitting the passenger in the next seat.

Get a cushy seat. Have you noticed that the middle seats often have more cushioning than the worn window and aisle seats? If they're velcroed on, get there early and exchange the seat cushions.

Window seats are for sleeping. If you're planning on getting a few zzz's, ask for a window seat so no one will be stepping over you. Grab a pillow and use earplugs and an eye mask. Inflatable u-shaped neck pillows are great too.

Survival tips for middle seats. If you're stuck in a middle seat, here are some survival tips. Claim both arm rests since your neighbors have more outside space and put your stuff in the overhead bin so you have more legroom. This is also a good time to close your eyes and practice meditation or read a small, paperback novel. Don't even try to use the computer or read a newspaper in this cramped space.

▶**Traveling is Expensive:**

- **Book your travel early.** Airline rates are usually the lowest at least three weeks out. But check out chapter nine's *References*, there are many last minute travel sites offering specials for travel on short notice.

- **Take a secondary airport.** Think about Midway instead of O'Hare, Burbank instead of LAX, and Love as an option to DFW. The secondary airports are often not only less expensive, but also easier to get in and out of.

- **Get the best deal.** Corporate hotel and car rental rates may not be the best deal. Ask if they are running any specials. If you don't already have a reservation, late evening hotel check-ins are generally more negotiable if they have rooms that may not sell otherwise. There have been times I've negotiated enough to have dinner for two "on the house." I carry an AAA (Automobile Association of America) card since the money I save on hotels greatly exceed the membership fee, plus they have great maps. AARP also offers nice discounts, but even if you're not a card-carrying member some hotels offer discounts to seniors.

- **Just ask.** If you have a frequent stay card with one hotel chain, but you're booked with another, ask if they'll give you a free upgrade to compare the two chains.

- **Ask others for recommendations.** Take advantage of your network of customers, friends, and people on your email listserve to find great, inexpensive places to stay and eat at your destination.

- **Save money on the exchange.** When traveling in a foreign country, get cash at an ATM machine, local bank, or use a credit card. These options provide the best exchange rates.

- **Use all your minutes.** I am provided a certain number of minutes on my cellular phone for a set price. If I go over, I pay more. But if I go under, it's my loss. If your plan is the same, ask your provider how to track the minutes used. If I'm well under my allotted free minutes near the end of my billing period, I start making personal and business calls from my mobile even when I'm at home. Why not take full advantage of the minutes you pay for anyway? Use them or lose them!

- **Save money on your phone bill.** Most frequent travelers have learned not to dial long-distance directly from the hotel phone. In addition to a possible connection fee, the minutes are often charged at operated-assisted rates or worse. If your hotel doesn't charge for toll free numbers, you may want use the phone for your long distance calls. If they *do* charge for toll-free numbers, I typically use my cell phone – especially when I still have plenty of minutes left. When using the internet, check with the front desk about local numbers for access with your internet provider. Don't assume just because you can get connected without dialing "1" that it a "local" call. You may be surprised at checkout when you get the bill.

- **Sign up for every frequent traveler program.** This is especially important when you don't have much control over the choices. At least you can get a free vacation every once in a while for all your troubles.

- **Don't tip twice.** Most hotels will automatically put a gratuity (often it's 17-20%) on your room service bill. Yet, they still leave a space for a "tip." Check it over carefully before you tip them twice.

▶**Cancellations Bum You Out?**

- **Check out the weather.** Use the internet, weather channel, or a newspaper to check the weather forecast before you leave home. In addition to your final destination, check the weather at your layover cities and final destination. If there are storms in the forecast, make some backup plans. If it's storming at home, allow plenty of time to get to the airport and check out alternate flights should your flight be delayed. If there's bad weather in your layover city, check on flights through another city. There have been times that I couldn't get to where I wanted that evening, but could get close. So

I just rented a car to drive the remainder. Bad weather at your final destination? Perhaps you'll want to make a reservation near the hotel and make the drive in the morning instead.

- **Take the best flight.** It's not always possible within our budget and our schedule, but keep in mind these tips. The first flight of the day more often leaves on time; as the day goes on there tends to be more delays. And, if you have an important meeting in the morning, never, never take the last flight out. Always allow at least one backup flight. If at all possible, travel on direct flights – even if it means not going on your favorite airline.

- **Note alternate flights.** When purchasing tickets, ask about earlier and later flights and alternate airlines that service your destination. Make a note of these options on your ticket jacket. If business plans change or there are delays due to equipment or weather, you'll be able to make backup plans quickly. If you fly mostly one airline, consider carrying their comprehensive flight guide with you.

- **Always confirm reservations** (hotel, air, limo) the day before travel. For international travel, confirm your return reservation at least 72 hours before your scheduled departure and again on the day before. To prevent being stranded, record the time, day, and the name of the agent who took your call.

- **Look forward to getting bumped.** Did you know that some travelers try real hard to get bumped? Why? Just for the free tickets or travel vouchers. I remember the time I got bumped from my inexpensive, two legged trip to New York and received a $500 airline voucher. In addition, they booked me first class on the next direct flight. I actually got there earlier than I would have on my original flight. What a deal! Another time, when I was connecting through my hometown of Houston, I got bumped. Again I got a travel voucher, a confirmation on the first flight the next morning, and the opportunity to surprise my family that evening. How can you get in on the action? As long as your schedule permits, leave earlier than you need to or purposely select a flight that is frequently overbooked. If the flight is oversold, the last ones checked in might be denied a seat. If you get to the airport early, request to be placed on the bump list. But don't forget to ask if you'll be confirmed on the next flight and if they'll pay for additional expenses such as hotel, food, and rental car.

- **Always have a back up.** If you go to the same city often, treat it like your second home. When meetings get cancelled, have a list of optional things to do along with phone numbers. In addition to work-related activities, you might consider getting a massage, manicure, teeth cleaning (perhaps they have a cancellation), a hair cut, a golf game, or just take a walk in a park.

- **Get in line and make your phone call.** If the flight gets cancelled or delayed, get on the mobile phone while you're waiting in line with all the other stranded souls. Call your travel agent or the airline directly (you'll find toll-free numbers in chapter nine). Chances are you'll find out what your options are before you make it to the ticket counter. Sometimes the changes can be made over the phone. Othertimes the agent will need to see the ticket, but at least you're better prepared with your options at hand. When a flight is delayed and they don't seem to know when (or if) it'll make it off the ground, try to book yourself on a later flight just in case this one doesn't make it.

- **Always guarantee your hotel room for a late arrival.** Even if you expect to be arriving early, it's best to guarantee your room with a credit card since travel plans often go awry.

How to Stay Healthy & Fit on the Road

▶**Tough Being Away From Home?** Sure it is. To make your visit more comfortable, be assertive about getting the best room possible. Have a good tip ready, but don't hand it to the bellman if the room doesn't meet your needs. If it has soiled carpeting, bad plumbing, or noisy neighbors, ask for another room. In addition:

- **Stick to the same 1 or 2 hotels** on each visit to the same city so you feel more at home.

- **Rent the same model of car**. That way you don't have to get out of the car to see which side has the gas tank or where the quick release tab is.

- **Maintain at least one daily ritual from home.** This provides you with one predictable rhythm. Perhaps that ritual will be your solitude or planning time, exercise routine, the times you get up and eat, or the foods you eat.

- **Make it feel like home.** As soon as you enter your hotel room, tuck all the hotel literature in a drawer and put out a framed picture of your loved ones that you packed from home. You might also consider carrying your own pillow or pillowcase, favorite pjs or sweats, or your favorite book. Give yourself a homey "olfactory fix" by lightly spritzing the pillowcases and towels in your hotel room with the same spray you use at home. Or just carry one of the dryer scent sheets you use in the dryer.

- **Do your laundry on the road.** So you can enjoy your time off when you return home, if you have the time, send out the dry cleaning or use the laundry room on-site so you can come home with clean clothes. If you're returning back to the same city after the weekend, leave your dry cleaning behind so it's ready when you return.

- **Don't forget to get your miles.** Then at least you'll be able to look forward to taking your family on an up-coming trip. Randy Petersen, editor of Inside Flyer, suggests keeping a checkbook for your frequent flyer miles. When you fly or engage in activities that accrue miles, enter the dates and other details. When you receive the credit, check them off. Place your ticket receipts in an envelope, write the date and connections on the front of the envelope, and file it under the airline – just in case the miles don't show up on your statement.

- **Find a stress-free hotel.** Take the ravel out of travel by selecting a hotel that caters to your needs. Which amenities do you find essential? A quick breakfast, good restaurant, safety, health facilities, business services, or plenty of movie channels? Consider in-room amenities such as: iron and board, hair dryer, coffee maker, easy-to-use alarm clocks, message services, or 24 hour room service (perhaps available by the pool).

- **Befriend the hotel personnel** especially on extended stays. It's nice to be greeted by a friend when you return from work or on your next trip. When you remember the names of key employees and ask about their families, they will become like extended family and will offer personalized service.

- **Take your loves ones with you.** Brainstorm about how you can take your family and friends along on a business trip so traveling and down time are more fun. Sometimes extra hands come in handy when you are carrying presentation materials or navigating unfamiliar cities. Although your dog can't help you carry things, some travelers take them along for companionship, safety, and as a reminder to exercise two or three times daily.

▶**Hate Waiting?** The average business traveler has hours of idle time. Our phone calls get placed on hold and we have to wait at the airport, in restaurants, and between appointments. Instead of getting angry (what good does that do?), use your idle time effectively. Here are some suggestions:

- **Read a book.** Keep a book in your carry-on and take along a reading light on a neck chain for dim-light situations such as on planes, buses, and limos.

- **Catch up on business reading.** I keep journals and other business-related reading in a pile in my office. When heading out of town, I grab a short stack on the

123

way out the door. If I don't need to keep them, it feels good to tear out the pages as I read them and come home with a lighter load. Or make notes as to what you need to do with each (put in database, call, file) so you can take care of it quickly when you return. Take advantage of the availability of magazines and newspapers on your travels for information on trends and your competitors. You might even come up with some great ideas for an upcoming presentation, solutions to a problem at work, or a list of things to do at your destination.

- **Listen to books on tape.** Instead of straining your eyes, consider listening to books-on-tape. You can find business, self-improvement, or fiction books-on-tape in your local library, grocery store, new and used bookstores, and through a variety of audiobook clubs.

- **Journal.** With nothing but a pen and pad of paper express your emotions and your thoughts. Traveling alone offers the perfect opportunity to become introspective and reflect on the little things that are the most important in your life or to release your anger.

- **Go to the airport chapel** or a secluded area for a moment of serenity in an otherwise hectic atmosphere.

- **Do something fun.** It could be as simple as looking at the scenery or visiting a toy shops. Bring along your needlepoint or another craft to keep your hands busy – and so you won't snack.

- **Create a travel diary.** Make travel an adventure by keeping notes of good hotels for future visits, museums or tourist sites to visit, and recommended restaurants.

- **Get something accomplished.** The night before you leave on a trip, write down the small things that need to be done. When you're waiting you can pay your bills, do your expense reports, read the backlog of emails, or place a call to the fix-it guy or to your child's school.

- **Learn something.** Listen to tapes or use a computer program to learn a second language, improve your keystroke speed, or brush up your math skills. Daily linguist (www.dailylinguist.com) is a free service to learn foreign languages. The site includes links to audio files for practicing pronunciation.

- **Shop specialty stores** for birthday, anniversary, and holiday gifts. Take advantage of the items found only in these parts of the country or world.
- **Use e-tickets.** Check-in is much faster.
- **Rent the car first, then get your checked luggage.** It saves you time and is convenient when the counter is in the same area and you can watch your luggage.
- **Drop off your luggage first.** Before returning your rental car, drop your luggage off curbside and check it. That way, after returning your car, you can just hop on the shuttle back to the airport unencumbered.

A Dozen Things to Do While Waiting in Line:

People watch. Kids are especially fun.

De-lint your outfit. Open up your expired bar-coded baggage label – it makes a great lint brush!

File your nails.

Brainstorm. Keep a running list of your worries. Jot down solutions (including the wildest) and eventually you'll come up with one that works.

Read.

Go shopping. Take your mail order catalogs with you and call in your order when you arrive.

Return a phone call.

Write a thank you note. Carry pre-stamped cards and envelopes and cards with you.

Listen to music or a book-on-tape.

Daydream. Why not?

Jot down notes. Pull out the business cards you've collected. Jot down notes and follow-up needed.

Plan your day. Or revamp your schedule.

▶**Hate Having to Catch Up When You Return?**

- **It's time to get a notebook computer.** Use your notebook computer to its full capacity. It's not just for word processing. Make sure you have a modem to fax and email. Your hotel front desk should have local access numbers for on-line services. If you travel internationally and want to take your laptop with you, hoping to stay connected on-line, you'll find this recent article, written by a PC World columnist, useful. It will help you prepare for your trip and save you some troubles and frustrations: http://www.resource-a-day.com/resources/stillonline.

- **Do two things at once.** Catch up on the news and your exercise at the same time. Brush your teeth and do some butt-busting lunges.

- **Have an in-box on the road.** On extended trips, have your assistant forward your mail via overnight delivery along with a pre-addressed overnight envelope to return it. During your down time on planes or when waiting, catch up on the paperwork and send it back to the office.

- **Bring your mail with you** if you don't have time to go through it. Discard the junk mail and then classify the remaining mail as urgent/important or can wait. Beginning with the important/urgent, review each, handle it, send off what you need to delegate, or document (use a post-it) what needs to be done when you return. No assistant? Carry prepaid overnight mail forms and envelopes with you so you can mail it back home or to the office.

- **Handle it immediately.** Keep track of travel expenses, and the related paperwork, on a day-to-day basis rather than waiting until you get home. Have you ever come home with business cards of people you don't remember meeting? Immediately after meeting someone, jot down (on the back of their business card) a note with information such as where you met, distinguishing features, phonetic spelling of their name, and what follow-up is needed. The same thing goes for phone calls and other important communication. Have to write a business report after your trip? As much as you'd like to get home right away, consider staying another night to finish up the work while the details are all still fresh in your mind, maximizing rest, and minimizing interruptions.

- **Use an off-airport parking service**. It's less expensive and often faster in peak times. Even better, some cities offer a parking service that will fill up your car, clean it, and do minor repairs and maintenance. That's one thing you can check off you weekend errand list.

Enjoy the Ride

Travel doesn't have to be all work and no play. There's an Old Chinese saying that "one joy dispels a hundred cares." Having a bit of fun everyday helps to clear your mind, regroup your thoughts, and mentally prepare yourself for the challenges that lay ahead – and makes you feel like you've had a mini vacation. But don't just expect to "find" the time, schedule some "me time" into every trip without feeling guilty. If the only fun thing you can think to do while traveling is to order dessert (did you know that "stressed" spelled backwards is "desserts"?), here are some other ideas:

▶**Do Something Different.** If you include enough of these ideas in your travels, you may actually look forward to traveling.

- **Order room service and watch a movie** – without interruption.
- **Read a fun book** that you allow yourself to read only on trips.
- **Go to the theatre**. Even when Broadway shows are "sold out," there are often single seats available.
- **Develop a hobby** that is best practiced on the road such as coin collecting, visiting historical places, or architectural design.

- **Enjoy the foods that you seldom eat at home.** For example, if everyone else in the family hates fish (but you love it), eat it out often on your travels.

- **Appreciate the little things.** Living in Texas makes me appreciate the freshly fallen snow on my trips – snow that I don't have to shovel.

- **Enjoy the luxury that travel can offer.** Sometimes it's just the little things like fresh flowers in the lobby, chocolates on the pillow, breakfast in bed, or a swim in the pool. Enjoy reading the morning news in the coffee shop or taking a walk along the flowering walkways. Maybe you have time to get a massage, manicure, or pedicure – guys, I'm talking about you too!

- **Go shopping.** Let's face it, you probably don't have time to shop when you're at home. When you have a block of time, shop for a special present for yourself and others, do your catalog shopping, or arrange for groceries to be delivered when you return. Since I can't find my favorite *Tetley*® tea at home, I search for it when I travel.

- **Change your mood.** Bring your own aromatherapy candles, oils, and sprays for your room. Energizing scents include spearmint, peppermint, pine, fir, spruce, lemon, basil, cardamon, and rosemary. Rose, lavender, chamomile, and sandalwood are considered relaxing scents. Vanilla elicits a positive outlook on life, while citrus is considered to lighten your mood and improve the immune system.

- **Visit your "peace corner."** Use your favorite music, relaxation tapes, or nature sounds to relax, meditate, or journal.

▶**Think About the Possibilities.** Approach travel with a positive, inquisitive attitude as if you were the ambassador. Talk to the locals, check out the architecture, and learn the history.

- **Do the Local Scene.** Satisfy your gypsy leanings through experiencing the local culture. Ask the taxi drivers, the concierge, and people you meet about the local museums, sporting events, restaurants, and entertainment.

- **See the sights.** Perhaps you have time to take a quick walk to the Liberty Bell, ride on a San Francisco trolley, or try some of the local foods. If you have more time, stay an extra day to take in a city tour or visit a nearby national park. Travel offers you the opportunity to see new sights, but not just at your final destination. Since there are often many ways to get there, think about routing your trip through a fun place. Perhaps there's a layover city that you've never visited – now's your time!

- **Meet up with friends and family.** It's fun to hook up with old friends who live near your destination or take a mini-vacation by inviting someone to accompany you.

- **Look for something positive.** Even when things don't go quite as you planned, be open to something interesting to come out of it. I remember when I flew to New York City to be interviewed on the Fox News Channel about my book, *Dining Lean*. Just hours before, the TV station called to reschedule the interview due to the escalating conflict in Bosnia. Since I was already in New York, I looked up an old high school girlfriend and had a blast catching up after more than 15 years. When your plans change, ask yourself what else you can do. If you're frequently passing through the same cities, consider packing a travel book which recommends good restaurants, hotels, sights to see and fun things to do just in case your plans fall through.

- **Have fun.** Looking for a new car? Instead of relying on just a test-drive, call the rental car companies to see if they have the vehicle for rent on an upcoming trip. Or rent something completely different to impress your clients or just have fun.

How to Stay Healthy & Fit on the Road

▶**Come Back Looking Younger.**

- **Take care of your personal care.** Make your hotel room your personal spa. Use your evenings to color your hair (guys too), pluck your eyebrows, or give yourself a facial. The hotel shower cap is perfect to deep condition your hair.

- **Take a hot bath** to erase the stress from your day. If you plan it right, you can start the tub when you arrive, order room service, unpack, take a soak, and be out when dinner is served and the movie starts. If you have wrinkled clothes, don't forget to hang them in the bathroom at the same time. (You may want to pack a few kitchen antiseptic cleaning cloths in a baggie to give the tub a rub down before making your bath.)

- **Exercise**. Besides being healthy for your heart, muscles and bones, exercise can also help you maintain your energy level and manage stress throughout a demanding day. Pamper yourself with a stretch, walk, or workout in the fitness center.

- **Laugh.** Laughing is an emotional exercise that builds up our immune system and helps to de-stress us. Look around on your trips for things to laugh about – like the silly things you do. Read the comics, the latest humor bestseller, or a book of jokes. Watch a comedy show or just watch people. Call a friend who always makes you laugh.

Have a safe trip!

Chapter 6

*Getting Your
Wheels in Gear*

In This Chapter:
▶Tips for Packing Light, Fast, and
  Wrinkle-Proof
▶Packing List of Essentials
▶*Dr Jo's Travel Favorites*

Every vehicle has a weight limit. What's yours? Probably less than you've been lugging around recently. While lifting weights at the gym may be healthy for you, hefting your overstuffed luggage is NOT. It's a good way to pull a muscle and add more tension to an already stressful trip. Frequent travelers have learned to pack as little as possible. Here are some tips on keeping your bags light:

Tips for Packing Light, Fast, and Wrinkle-Proof

▶ **Lighten Your Load.** My husband went on his first international business trip a decade ago. Planning an eight day trip day to Italy, France, and England, he stuffed eight outfits into this huge suitcase. When he arrived at the Venice train station, he was informed that the hotel was a quarter

131

mile away – and there was no transportation! After that trip, he vowed never to travel without wheels and to never carry more than he needed. For your next trip:

- **Make it a roll-on.** Roll-on luggage makes dashing about easier and is healthier for your back. Look for padded, adjustable height handles; inline skating wheels that are smooth and quiet; and a strap to attach a briefcase or second bag. If you frequently need to lug around your briefcase without the assistance of a wheeled suitcase, consider buying a briefcase with wheels, one that converts into a backpack (www.swissarmy.com), or carrying a small luggage cart (www.Magellans.com).

- **Make it light weight.** Start off with a lightweight, soft-sided case rather than a heavy hard-sided one.

- **Consider only carry-on luggage.** Whether it's a five day business trip or a two week vacation, it's possible to pack all your essentials in one carry-on bag. You'll never have to worry about lost luggage or endure waiting at the baggage terminal. Airline regulations allow you to carry-on a bag up to 22" X 9" X 14."

- **Consider the features you need.** Hanging valets enable compact packing for suits. Zippered pockets help to keep items separated and easy-to-find and are a great place for dirty clothes. Outside pockets are useful for items you need at the airport or during the flight. What features do you need?

- **Pack as little as possible.** Frequent travelers have learned to travel light. Unless you'll be seeing the same client everyday, you can get away with wearing the same clothes more than one day. The secret comes in selecting comfortable, travel-friendly, washable, wrinkle-resistant clothing that mix and match with each other. More on this later.

▶ **Plan Ahead.** Before you leave town, here are some things to consider:

- **At home, keep your bag permanently packed.** Frequent flyers take the ravel out of travel by keeping some items permanently packed in their suitcase. This may include items such as your toilet bag, workout clothes, sleep wear, umbrella, undergarments, and business shoes. As soon as you return from your trip, replace the used items. When business or pleasure calls again, all you have to do is add those few pieces of clothing and you're ready to leave on your next trip.

- **Keep a packing list.** Have you ever panicked on the way to the airport because you had forgotten (or thought you had forgotten) something? Avoid the unnecessary stress by keeping a packing list on the computer. I have different lists for: a short business trip, longer business trip, trip to the beach, or a ski trip. Oh, and don't forget to put "airline ticket" on your list. I am so accustomed to using e-tickets that once, when a client sent me paper tickets, I forgot them at the office. Since I didn't have time to pick them up, I had to buy another ticket. Ouch!

- **Get ready.** As you approach your departure day, start collecting things you'll need. Keep a file, box, or your open briefcase in your office. As it occurs to you, toss in your tickets, maps, phone numbers, client files, and reading materials you're going to bring on the trip. But don't forget to double-check against your packing list.

- **Do it in miniature.** Don't waste space with full-size versions of your deodorant, shampoo, and lotions. Bring sample sizes or decant them into mini-bottles (www.containerstore.com has a large variety). Screw-on pill bottles (I've found some of the snap-ons open accidentally) are also a great way to carry a few of your most needed pain relievers, antihistamines, and other medications. They're also a good way to store q-tips, cotton balls, safety pins, and jewelry – or use disposable camera film containers.

133

- **Think double duty.** When purchasing travel items, think about getting those items that will serve multiple purposes. For example, there are clothes steamers that also boil water. Ladies can pack an oversized t-shirt that can be used for sleeping and as a pool cover-up. Consider a sports watch with an alarm instead of packing an extra alarm clock. My favorite *TravelSmith® CoolMax®* workout shirt is nice enough to wear under a suit in a pinch. The Lite II (www.containerstore.com) contains folding scissors, eyeglass screwdriver, file, staple puller, tweezers, tooth pick, and six other functions in a card not much bigger than a credit card.
- **Buy lightweight.** In addition to lightweight luggage, go for the lightweight raincoat, suit, and accessory bag.
- **Use clear bags.** Although you can buy small zippered cloth bag, I use plastic zip-lock freezer bags. Place undergarments in one and socks in another. How about a third for cosmetics and lotions? They're transparent, inexpensive, and spills are contained.
- **Suck out the air.** Many stores carry specialty bags that, as you roll them up, literally suck the air out. Although clothes wrinkle badly, the system is good for packing bulky items such as your pillow, ski bibs, sweaters, fleece clothing, and dirty laundry. Look for names like *PacMates, Pack-it®* and *Travel Space Bags*.

▶ **Travel in Comfort.** There was a day when a road trip or flight meant getting decked out in our Sunday best – stiff, uncomfortable clothing that we couldn't wait to get off. Unless you're being met at the airport by a client, it's OK to dress for comfort – but that doesn't mean bumming it.

- **Travel casual.** Select an outfit you can conduct business in if your luggage gets lost or your flight is delayed and there's no time to change. This might include a pair of slacks (no jeans) and jacket or sweater or perhaps a classy two piece workout suit. Layering is a good idea since the temperature can range from stifling hot before takeoff to arctic freeze once the air is turned on.

- **Wrinkle-resistant, comfortable clothes.** So you don't look like you slept in your clothes (even if you did), consider elastic waists and wrinkle-resistant, stretchy fabrics. Pick colors and styles that mix and match with the clothes you've packed. Stay away from tight socks or knee high stockings that cut off your circulation.

- **Flat, comfortable walking shoes.** Let's face it, they're more comfortable than your dress shoes. Keep a pair just for travel purposes so they stay newer looking and clean. I travel in my running shoes so I don't need to pack a third pair. You're going to workout, aren't you?

- **A front-worn shoulder bag or fanny pack.** As you'll see in the *Passing the Safety Inspection* chapter, it's safer to carry essential items in your front pockets. If you must have a bag, select one that leaves your hands free to carry the luggage. While a backpack or large shoulder bag may be comfortable, it's also easy for a thief to access. Scale down so you can carry as little as possible in a fanny pack or small shoulder bag worn in the front of your body. More and more men are wearing fanny packs because of the comfort and convenience.

▶ **Simplify Your Clothes.** Here are some tips to keep your clothing to a minimum:

- **Buy washable, travel-friendly, wrinkle-free clothing.** Save yourself the time of ironing or steaming by buying only wrinkle-resistant (or even wrinkle-proof) clothing. Stay away from most natural fibers such as 100% cotton or linen. If you like cotton, look for shirts that are 60% cotton, 40% polyester. They're breathable and comfortable, yet don't wrinkle as badly as 100% cotton. Or look for the new blend of cotton with 3-5% *lycra*® in shirts, pants, and jackets – they stretch for comfort, are more wrinkle-resistant, yet look like cotton. Other fabrics that hold up well to travel include wool, triacetate, good quality silks, cashmere sweaters, microfiber, fleece, microfleece, and polyester. Other wrinkle-free, breathable fabrics include *Supplex*®,

135

CoolMax®, *Lycra®*, and *Primaloft®*. When shopping, give the clothes the wrinkle test before you buy – crush the fabric in your hand and release. If it's full of wrinkles, don't buy it! You don't want to spend your evenings ironing, do you?

- **Pack a minimum number of outfits**. You can usually get away with fewer business suits than the number of days on your trip. So you don't look like you're wearing the same outfit, pack a different shirt or blouse for each day. At least one should be a neutral colored, quick-dry, washable shirt or shell (such *CoolMax®* or washable silk) that can be washed in the hotel sink and worn again if your trip gets extended. Even for a two week vacation, you can get by with three bottoms, three tops, and three vests/sweaters/jackets if you select those that mix and match with each other.

- **Keep to one color scheme.** It's best to pick from black, navy, brown, and olive since they're professional-looking, don't show dirt easily, and match with so many other colors. By sticking to one color scheme on each trip you'll reduce your need for extra accessories like ties, belts, purses, and jewelry.

- **Pack just one pair of dress shoes.** Another reason to select just one color scheme, is that you need just one pair of dress shoes – one of the heaviest and bulkiest items in your bag. Buy shoes you can comfortably walk in all day long (no high heels ladies). To minimize space, pack socks into your shoes instead of using shoe horns. Wrap shoes in plastic grocery bags or flannel shoe bags (www.Magellans.com) to keep your clothes clean and your shoes scratch-free. Pack shoes and other heavy items on the bottom of the suitcase so the load doesn't end up top-heavy.

- **Select all-season clothing.** Consider investing in suits that are comfortable all year long (or at least three seasons). That way, when you're traveling to both warm and cold climates on the same trip, you won't need to pack two different suits – just pack a turtleneck and a short sleeved shirt. Instead of a winter coat, invest in a high quality, wrinkle resistant, lightweight all-weather coat with zip-in lining – preferably one that is washable.

- **Add coordinating colors.** Basic suits can be jazzed up with colorful shirts, ties, scarves, sweaters, and jewelry in coordinating colors.

▶ **Pack Right.** If you buy wrinkle-resistant clothing, packing is easy – just fold them neatly. If you don't want to invest in wrinkle-resistant clothing, here are some tips to make them look their best:

- **Wrap in plastic.** Place each item of clothing in a plastic dry cleaner bag, stack up to six items, and then fold in thirds smoothing out air pockets as you go.
- **Get your dress shirts folded at the dry cleaner.** They'll pack better (and come out looking better) than hanging them or folding them yourself.
- **Iron it.** Don't pack an iron. Even if you need one, most US hotels (and abroad) have irons in the hotel rooms or are available upon request.
- **Turn on the steam.** Leave the steamer at home too. Just turn on the shower as hot as it will go, hang your clothes where they won't get wet, close the door, and leave them until the wrinkles are gone. Clipping a skirt hanger onto the bottom of your outfit helps to pull out wrinkles.
- **Dryer sheet minimizes static.** You know those sheets that you throw in the dryer to minimize wrinkles? Keep one in an open plastic bag in your luggage to keep clothes smelling fresh. It can be rubbed against the inside of an outfit or hair to eliminate static cling.

Packing List of Essentials

▶ **Permanently Packed Items.** While each of us will have a different packing list, the following items offer you some ideas (please, don't pack them all) of what to keep permanently packed at all times. Just add your clothes and you're ready to go.

☐ **Toilet Bag.** Since counter space may be limited, consider a bag that will sit *or* hang on a hook, towel rack, or shower rod. If you don't want to buy duplicates of everything at home, keep the bag next to your sink, always restocked and ready to go. Put a small golf pencil and index card in the bag to jot down what you're getting low on. Restocking the bag can then be done without doing a complete inventory of your bag. Your bag may include:

Deodorant, moisturizer, lotion, lip balm, make-up
Razor (Magellan has a retractable one), steptic pencil
Toothbrush, toothpaste, dental floss
Tissues, individually wrapped antibacterial handwipes
Pain relievers, antihistamines, and other needed pills
Antacids, vitamin/mineral supplements
Bandaids and/or blister protectors
Few pieces of jewelry/cufflinks that go with everything
Comb or foldable brush/mirror

☐ **Undergarments.** Invest in some quick dry undergarments (see www.TravelProducts.com or www.travelsmith.com). If your trip goes longer than expected, you can handwash them in the sink. Ladies, for longer trips carry plenty of panty liners. In a pinch, they can keep you fresh in lieu of changing panties. They're also useful for incontinence problems. And don't forget to pack extra pantyhose.

☐ **Business shoes.** Remember, just one pair.

☐ **Sleepwear.** Consider a microfiber set that isn't bulky. Silk long johns are not only great for sleeping, if the weather turns unexpectedly cold or the convention hall puts the air conditioning on overdrive, you can slip them under your suit (available in shorties to wear with a dress). Microfiber sleepwear and silk long johns are both available at www.Magellans.com and www.TravelSmith.com.

138

☐ **Workout clothes**. Bring just one set of workout clothing in the new quick-dry, breathable materials such as *Supplex®*, *CoolMax®*, and *Tactel®*. After working out, just hop in the shower with your clothes on, wring them out, and then hang them up to dry. Consider these:

Shorts and shirt (one of each)
Sneakers (make these your travel shoes)
Quick dry bathing suit and goggles
Packable lightweight rain suit to workout in the rain
Fleece jacket, stretch pants, gloves & hat for cold weather

☐ **Lightweight, aluminum umbrella.**

▶ **Other Things to Consider.** Here are some other things you may want to pack.

☐ **Lightweight rain coat with zip-in lining**. Some travelers bring just a foldable poncho. A bungee cord is useful to attach your coat to your luggage when trudging through the airport.

☐ **Gloves.** If there's even a slight chance for cold-weather, tuck in a pair of light-weight gloves. I always carry a pair of polypropylene gloves (www.rei.com). These washable gloves are great for an early morning jog or when the cold weather sneaks up on you.

☐ **Collapsible bag.** A sturdy, zippered, lightweight, collapsible bag is useful to bring fruit back from the market or to collect souvenirs along the way. Accumulate your dirty clothes in the bag and check it on the return trip as an additional piece of luggage. When you return home there's no need to sort out your dirty clothes.

☐ **Flat slippers.** Slippers that pack flat can be worn to the pool and in the shower. Keep the free sock slippers you get on international flights; they make great shoe covers.

☐ **Ziploc baggies.** Pack a few of both the small and gallon-sized ones. These will come in handy for everything from carrying wet clothes, business receipts, or saving a roll leftover from room service.

139

How to Stay Healthy & Fit on the Road

☐ **Kitchen kit.** If you're packing your own food, like those mentioned in *Fueling the Engine* chapter, pack a heating coil; plastic, thermal mug; small, plastic plate, and utensils (www.Magellans.com has a SnacPac Picnic set of a fork, knife, and spoon that neatly stashes together).

☐ **Alarm.** If you consider your destination unsafe, pack a small security alarm and/or motion detector that connect to the hotel door or the locked sleeping compartment on the train.

☐ **A "bring-me-back something" gift for kids.** Sure it's fun to search for that special gift, but if you run out of time to shop on your trip, you'll have a back-up. There are plenty of gift ideas in the *Staying Balanced* chapter.

☐ **Traveler's convenience items.** If you'll be doing a lot of reading in your hotel room, the usual 60 watt hotel light bulb is inadequate. You could take your own 100 watt light bulb (some people actually do) or get a portable light that is worn around your neck for low-lit places. Other items include a surge protector, telephone extension cord so you can use the phone anywhere, and plug converters when traveling abroad. When we go on motor home vacations, we each pack our own *Aquis®* towels (www.Brookstone.com carry them). These quick dry towels soak up a lot of water, take up very little space, and dry many times faster than regular towels.

☐ **Pleasure items.** If you miss some of the luxuries and comfort of home, pack a few pleasure items like bubble bath, bath salts, an inflatable bath pillow, candles, incense, aromatic oil, folding fan for hot climates, or a picture from home. You may also consider packing a portable CD or tape player with your favorite tunes, a relaxation tape, or a book on tape.

☐ **Large scarf.** Ladies, pack a large scarf to cover your head when traveling abroad (especially when visiting churches). It also comes in handy as a quick exercise or pool cover-up, briefcase concealer, bad hair day camouflage, or to dress up an outfit.

☐ **Emergency kit.** Consider taking a mini flashlight for blackouts, emergency retreats from hotels, and middle of the night bathroom visits. Duct tape also comes in handy to repair glasses, a broken strap, loose hem, or broken zipper. Just wrap a foot or two around a pencil or popsicle stick. Hotels don't always have enough skirt hangers, so you may want to pack your own. Pack a couple of clothes pins for closing drapes when needed.

☐ **Laundry kit.** If you're packing a lot of washable clothing, consider packing your own laundry soap in a small bottle (I just use shampoo), a sink stopper (many hotels out of the country don't have one), and spot remover.

▶ **What to Take in Your Briefcase or Purse.** If it's difficult to find what you need or to fit it all in your briefcase, it's time to lighten your load. Consider these:

☐ **Paper or electronic organizer/address book.** Scale your organizer down as small as possible. A personal digital assistant such as Palm (www.palm.com) or Handspring (www.handspring.com) organizers carry more information and are much lighter than paper organizers. Leave your frequent flyer and frequent stayer cards behind if just having the number in your organizer will do. And pack just one pen and one pencil.

☐ **Wallet.** To reduce the weight in your fanny pack or purse, keep coins in your pocket and carry just paper money and travelers checks in your wallet. Leave your frequent shopper cards, library cards, and department cards at home. Since checks are often not accepted outside your hometown, leave them behind as well. Trim down to just one business and one personal credit card – preferably those that offer low interest rates, travel mileage, or a rebate. If you were to lose your wallet or purse, you'll be glad you had just a couple to cancel. And narrow your pictures down to just a couple. Now that you've trimmed down the contents, you may be able to leave the wallet and use just a money clip, velcro strap, or rubber band to carry the essentials in your front pocket.

How to Stay Healthy & Fit on the Road

☐ **Cellular phone and/or pager.** Travelers often find cellular phones indispensable especially when there's a line for the phone, you're late or lost, or your car breaks down. If your flight gets cancelled you can call the airline while you're waiting in line at the customer service center, touch base with family and clients while you're in a taxi, and depending on your plan, it can save you money over long distance connection fees. Don't forget your phone charger, car adapter, and a hands-free/voice activated phone system.

☐ **Water.** Keep bottles of frozen water in your home freezer that you can grab on your way out the door. It's less expensive than buying it at the airport and easier than waiting for the drink cart. By the time your flight takes off, it'll be melted but still cold.

☐ **Eyeglasses.** Pack your eyeglasses or sunwear in a padded case that has a clip. When you're walking without your briefcase or purse, you can clip them to your belt.

☐ **Sleeping aids.** When you want to catch some zzz's, carry foldable eye shades, foam or silicone ear plugs, an inflatable neck pillow (for comfort, don't overinflate) and a pair of compact slippers for your resting comfort.

☐ **Essentials bag.** If you've checked your luggage, tuck some essentials into your briefcase. These may include an extra shirt, undergarment, pantyhose, toothbrush, toothpaste, tissues, and individually wrapped handiwipes (www.herbanessentials.com, 888-320-6994 has some nice scented ones). To make the flight more comfortable, consider lubricating eye drops, moisturizer, saline nose spray, chewing gum, and a decongestant nose spray (consult your doctor first).

☐ **Business kit.** Take business cards and notecards for quick thank yous. For a small office-to-go check out www.travelproducts.com – theirs contains 10 frequently used items including a ruler, stapler, scissors, and pen. I also bring post-its, floppy disks, highlighter, and a legal pad. You may also want to add self-stick address labels or an address stamper if you're often asked to fill out contact information (such as at conventions). Large envelopes for collecting receipts or sending completed work home or expense reports to the home office also come in handy. Don't forget extra batteries for your tape player, computer, and cell phone.

☐ **Camera.** Although vacationers usually pack a camera, business people might also want to tuck a disposable camera in their briefcase. There are always opportunities to photograph something touristy, clients, or special events. Giving pictures to clients, along with a brief note is always a nice touch. The FAA recommends not carrying unprocessed film in a checked bag – the new explosives detection systems might leave a foggy half-inch streak on the film. Place it in your carry-on instead. Travel stores have X-ray bags that help to safeguard your memories.

☐ **Itinerary, maps, and contact information.** When traveling out of the country, include contact information for the US Embassy, maps, translation guides, and some local cash currency.

▶ **Getting Back Home:**

• **Mail it home.** Instead of carrying home the bulky seminar literature, souvenirs, or even dirty laundry that you accumulate along the way, use the hotel's concierge to send it home. Don't forget to mail things ahead to your destination as well.

• **Leave your clothes behind.** If you frequent the same city within a month's time, consider leaving your clothes at the cleaners. When you return, you'll have clean clothes ready for you. Remember to check the cleaner's "hold" policy and leave a phone number with them. You can also leave some nonessentials in the hotel storeroom.

• **Throw it away.** If you'll be roughing it on a camping trip and want to come back with lighter bags than when you left, pack up some of your older tees and undergarments. Then just trash them at the end of your trip.

143

Dr Jo's Travel Favorites
(company web sites and contact info are listed in chapter 9)

Raincoat – *TravelSmith®* wins hands down as my favorite raincoat – both in men's and ladies. It's lightweight, waterproof, and offered in a variety of colors and styles. The nearly weightless optional liner is surprisingly warm.

Umbrella – *Magellan's®* has the lightest, flat-packing umbrella. At 6oz, it's half as light as the other "lightweight" ones. Folded, it's about 1"X7".

Business Suit – If you're looking for a travel-friendly business suit, check out *TravelSmith®*'s Ladies Classic Travel Blazer and Trousers. They are comfortable, flattering, and have more options. You can select from: navy or black, pleated or plain pants, and short and long blazers. My husband, Lorin, favors *LLBean®*'s Microfiber Blazer and Pants. The blazer is offered in black and navy; pants come in plain, pleated, and hidden-comfort.

Dress Shirts – My husband and I prefer the comfort of silk shells and *CoolMax®* shirts when we're traveling. They're great-looking, wrinkle-resistant, non-bulky, washable, quick drying, and extremely breathable. My favorite is *TravelSmith®*'s Perfectly Packable Silk Tee. Lorin likes *TravelSmith®*'s CoolMax® button-down Travel Shirts (they look just like his other dress shirts) and *Magellan's®* Four-Season Silk Blend Tees.

Travel Dress – Nearly every catalog carries travel dresses that are wrinkle resistant – and is often offered in just black or navy. I chose *Land's End®* because of its flattering fit, variety of styles, and the wider variety of colors offered.

Travel Outfit – My favorite travel outfit is *Magellan's®* 2 piece navy travel suit. It's classy, as comfortable as sweats, and wrinkle-resistant. My husband wishes they made it in men's.

Dr Jo's Travel Favorites (cont.)

Casual Pants - My husband, when he's not wearing a suit, travels in his favorite *TravelSmith®* Kenya nylon convertible pants. They're nicely tailored, wrinkle-resistant, washable, quick-drying, and zipper off to become shorts. Even when I'm speaking, I tend to wear a funky blazer with one of my great-fitting, comfortable *Land's End®*'s Stretch Chinos. *Land's End®* is the only place I've found where I can specify a petite rise and tall inseam at no additional cost. The 5% *Lycra®* spandex in the otherwise cotton pants keeps them nearly wrinkle-free.

Casual Shirts - My husband has many *NorthFace®* button-down shirts in a variety of colors. They're comfortable, breathable, washable, and quick-drying. You can find a local retailer at www.NorthFace.com.

Fanny Pack – Even men are opting for the convenience of wearing a fanny pack. My favorites include both the small and large security waist packs available through *Magellan's®* or *TravelSmith®* Available in a luxuriously wonderfully soft leather or microfiber, each have a stainless steel cable built into the strap.

Workout Clothes – Our favorite workout tops are *CoolMax®* tee shirts from *TravelSmith®*. Unlike other *CoolMax®* shirts tested, *TravelSmith®*'s are substantial, not shear. For workout shorts and pants, my favorites are *Moving Comfort®* (made just for women).

Bathing Suit – *Land's End®* has a huge selection of ladies bathing suits to fit every shape and preference. Their Tugless Tanks are conservatively cut and quick-dry. However, ever since college swim team, I've bought *Speedo®* suits. My husbands's favorite is a pair of quick-dry *Speedo®* swim shorts.

Dr Jo's Travel Favorites (cont.)

Fleece – The whole family packs fleece jackets and pants for just about any cold-weather trip. These light, fluffy clothes are warm and very quick-drying. They shed water easily and are offered in many colors and fashionable styles including wind-proof styles that are incredibly warm. Most of our fleece (and microfleece) come from *LL Bean*®.

Suitcase – When I first began traveling in 1994, I did the research and selected a *Briggs & Riley*® ballistic nylon, wheeled carry-on. It's lightweight, extremely durable (I'm still using the same one), and fairly inexpensive. My husband and daughter both have their own *Briggs & Riley*® bags.

Briefcase – I love my *Swiss Army*® *Webmaster*™ – a ballistic nylon briefcase that offers the ultimate in functionality and organization. It has a removable laptop sleeve, an expandable main storage compartment, and an *outside* mesh pocket for my water bottle. And only *Swiss Army*® offers a $1500 laptop theft insurance policy (at no cost and with no deductible) with purchase and registration.

Chapter 7

Passing the Safety Inspection

In This Chapter:
▶Keeping You & Your Belongings Safe
▶Traveling Outside the Country
▶Medical Safety Tips

Although airplane crashes, tourist kidnappings, and murders make the headlines, you are far more likely to have your home robbed while you are away, suffer Montezuma's Revenge (traveler's diarrhea), or get pick-pocketed on your travels. While none of these incidences can be completely prevented, this chapter provides guidelines to help you stay safe on your travels.

Keeping You and Your Belongings Safe

The 1999 United States (US) Crime Index reports a rate of 4266.8 incidences of crime per 100,000 inhabitants. That's a yearly incidence rate of just 0.04%. Violent crimes make up 12% of the incidences while property crimes account for the other 88%. Although there are no solid statistics, it's been estimated that crimes against tourists are twice as high as crimes against locals.

That may be on the low side. A 1997 study by the Australia Bureau of Tourism Research found that of the 2840 visitors interviewed at the Sydney airport before they left the country, 2.3% had experienced harassment, an actual/attempted/threatened assault, robbery, or theft. That's extremely high considering that the average visit was just four days! Yet, interestingly, none of the harassments or assaults and only half of the thefts were even reported to the police.

Why are travelers more often victimized? Travelers have a higher visibility as a result of differences in their dress, speech, and behavior. Travelers also have certain personal and behavioral attributes that tend to make them *"desirable"* victims. They tend to carry larger sums of money and expensive jewelry and cameras. Travelers have also, unknowingly, wandered into areas that local residents tend to avoid.

This chapter provides suggestions on how to make yourself a less desirable victim. Although some of the tips may be considered common sense, they have been included because as Steven Covey says: "common sense isn't always common practice." Admittedly, you won't need to comply to all of the recommendations all of the time. We often hear crime victims say that they had a bad feeling prior to the incident, but had ignored their instincts thinking they were being silly. When it comes to our personal safety, I think it's important to heed our instincts – it's better to be safe than sorry.

▶ **Be Aware! Be Alert!** That's the motto of Pam Nimitz DeMaris, personal safety/crime prevention expert and web author of ithesurvivor.com. When you're talking to others, looking at a map, or preoccupied with your luggage, it's easy for the thief to take advantage of the situation. Here are a few examples of how to stay alert:

- **Don't become alcohol-impaired.** Alcohol impairs your thinking and lowers your guard. Being slipped the "date rape" drug in a drink or food is a much publicized risk for women. But men are also being drugged and robbed.

That's why it's always a good idea to drink with a known companion who can look out for you.

- **Be aware of your surroundings at all times.** When walking, keep alert of people, cars, doorways, stairwells, and the direction you are walking. Always have a plan in case you get into a dangerous situation.

- **On the plane, count the number of seats to the nearest exit.** And, when you're in your seat, keep your seatbelt buckled. They don't give you a warning light when you hit an air pocket or turbulence.

▶ **Don't Get Distracted.** We had just landed in Barcelona, Spain. Although we were tired from flying all night, our family checked into the hotel and took a walk up the hill to the site of the 1992 Summer Olympics.

Just a mile or so from the downtown hotel, we passed a well-dressed, young man walking in the opposite direction. He politely stopped us to inform us there was something on our clothing. Sure enough, although my husband had it the worst, the back of our pants were splattered with what looked like vomit. "Eww. Yuk." Although our grasp of Spanish was not much more than the basics, we understood that he wanted to help.

While I was attending to my six year old daughter's clothing, he reached in his pocket and opened a brand new bottle of water, pulled out some paper towels, and offered to assist my husband by cleaning the back of his pants. Just seconds later my husband picked up Alexandra, grabbed my hand, and ordered me to start running.

When we returned to the hotel we found it this was a common robbery scam. Working in teams, one group discreetly sprays the back of a tourist with chocolate milk, mustard, or another nasty looking substance. A bit later, the accomplice approaches with a bottle of water and some paper towels and offers to help clean the pants. It wasn't until the man

149

reached into my husband's back pocket that my husband realized what was happening. Fortunately, my husband carries his wallet in his zippered front pocket when traveling. We escaped without harm or loss, but the incident reinforced the importance of taking caution in every situation. To reduce your odds of being victimized by a thief:

- **Watch your luggage at security.** Don't walk through the metal detector until your luggage enters the machine on the security conveyor belt. If someone cuts through, tell them firmly that you're next. A common scam is for someone to hold up the line by intentionally setting off the metal detector while your luggage gets picked up at the other end. If you're traveling with another person, let them go ahead to collect the carry-ons while you make sure they make it through the belt. If security wants to search one of your bags, collect all your belongings before you submit to the search.

- **Keep your hands on your bag.** While someone is asking you directions and you use your hands to point, the second person can make off with your bag.

- **Be cautious if your car needs repairs.** Be weary of people who point out car problems. Thieves may intentionally puncture your tire at a rest stop and then motion you off the road. They may even help you change the tire while another party makes off with your valuables. Sometimes there is nothing wrong with your car, but they make you think that there is. Always keep your gas tank at least half full, windows shut, and check your tires to be sure they are fully inflated. If you get a flat, it's may be safer to ride the rim to the next exit or carry a can of *Fix-A-Flat®* instead of stopping to change the tire.

- **Keep your windows shut.** In high crime areas, hijackers can easily take advantage of an open window in a slow moving vehicle.

- **Be aware of the wrong change scam.** I recommend keeping a small currency converter handy so you don't ever get the wrong change. It's real easy for someone to

150

"accidentally" give you change for 10,000 lire instead of 100,000.

- **Be more cautious in crowds.** Bands of vagrant kids begging or selling goods often take advantage of large crowds on subways, in the market, or at a festival to pick your pocket or slice your purse or knapsack.

▶**Choose Safe Accommodations.**

- **Valet your car.** Particularly late at night, pay the extra few bucks to avoid the inherent risk of the dark parking lot or garage.

- **Select a hotel, not a motel.** Hotel rooms open to the interior of the building and often have cameras covering the few entrances. Motel rooms are open to the outside and are easy access for a thief.

- **Get a safe room.** A first floor room is more likely to have a break-in from the outside. A room very high up (over the sixth floor) can be more dangerous in a fire. Consider asking for a room that is closer to the elevator so you don't have a long walk down the hall.

- **Check the room to be sure it is vacant and secure.** When initially entering the room, prop the door open and check the room to ensure it is vacant. Make sure windows, adjoining doors, and sliding glass doors are locked. Check under the bed and behind the shower curtain. If everything is OK, put out the "Do not disturb" sign, close the door, and lock the deadbolt right away.

- **Do a room check upon arrival.** Familiarize yourself with the emergency escape route – which is often posted on the back of the door. To save yourself from having to call maintenance later, do a quick room check: make sure the hairdryer and telephone are working, shower and sink are draining properly, and the toilet doesn't run after it's flushed. Check for adequate hangers, towels, and toilet paper.

- **Follow the same safety rules that you tell your chil-**

151

dren. Never open your hotel room door without knowing who is there. If they announce that they are from maintenance, call the front desk to confirm before letting them in. Some travelers attach a personal alarm to the hotel door which sounds when the door is opened. Others use a simple rubber door jam or prop a glass or ash tray against the door.

- **Create the illusion of an occupied room.** When you leave your room, post the "Do Not Disturb" sign and leave the TV and some lights on so a potential intruder will think someone is in the room.

- **Take your valuables with you.** When staying in a hostel or other shared arrangement, take your valuables with you to the bathroom.

- **Call security if your neighbors are causing a disturbance.** To avoid possible altercations, don't play policeman. Instead of pounding on the wall or door, call security to handle the situation.

- **If it doesn't feel safe, go elsewhere.** Travelers generally make hotel reservations sight unseen. If, once you arrive, it doesn't feel right, go elsewhere. Even if it's after the 6pm check-in and you refuse payment, your credit card company will often work with you.

- **Have a flashlight handy.** While traveling, keep a small, high-powered flashlight on your nightstand in case of an emergency. Put your valuables in your purse and have it handy with your coat and shoes in the event of a fire alarm in the middle of the night.

▶ **Don't Stand Out.** On my first trip abroad we visited Italy's Amalfi Coast. It didn't take long to realize that even without opening my mouth (I don't speak Italian), everyone knew I was an American. How? After landing in Rome, we drove the short distance to Sorrento and took a walk along the beach. In every direction I looked, people were dressed in dark colored clothing with dark shoes. Silly me! I had worn a silky red, purple, and gold workout suit with white sneakers. Since crime is often focused on the foreigner, it's helpful to keep a low profile so you don't stand out. Consider these tips:

- **Avoid bright colored clothing.** Dark colored, especially black, clothing is always a better choice even for shoes. In some areas, it is recommended that you dress down and not wear a business suit.

- **Leave your expensive jewelry at home.** In addition, to wearing costume jewelry consider replacing an elaborate wedding set with a simple gold band when traveling out of the country. Single women visiting in male-dominated foreign countries may want to invest in a simple wedding ring to ward off unwanted male attention.

- **Don't flash your money**. When walking around town, carry just the minimum needed. Leave the rest in the hotel safe. Keep change handy for tipping or bus or subway fare so you don't have to reveal the contents of your wallet.

- **When renting a car, choose one with the license plate from the state you are in.** Otherwise people will know you're a visitor.

- **Familiarize yourself with the area.** You can always tell the tourist – they've got their head buried in a map. To avoid standing out, familiarize yourself with the area and get detailed directions – before you head out. If you get lost driving, head to a safe-looking store and ask for directions. If you're on a walking tour, you might want to jot down directions on a small piece of paper so you don't get distracted by continually looking at the map.

▶ **Protect Yourself and Your Identity.**

- **Minimize who knows you're gone.** Leave your itinerary with family or friends so they know how to get in touch with you. But since most homes are robbed when there's no one home, do you really need to advertise it on your home recorder or voice mail?

153

- **Don't advertise your home address.** Since your mail and magazines have your home address on them, don't just leave them lying around at restaurants and hotels without first ripping off the address label.
- **Use laminated business card as luggage tags**. These should have your *business* address and phone number rather than your home information.
- **Don't tell new acquaintances on the plane your final destination.** You never know who might be listening in on your conversation.
- **Protect confidential information.** It's best to wait until you're in the privacy of your hotel room or office to review your confidential information. Remember that even if your seatmates aren't looking, the person behind you on the plane may still be able to read your computer screen.
- **Present your business card when checking in**. To avoid having to verbally announce your name, address, and phone number, give them a business card to copy.
- **Do not allow your room number to be announced**. If they do verbally give out the room number, ask for another room.
- **Make hotel and restaurant reservations using just your last name** and the first initial of your first name.
- **Protect crucial information.** When punching in PIN numbers or your credit card information, use your hand and body to block view. Thieves have been known to use binoculars to steal numbers. Don't allow hotel chains to use your social security number as their membership number.

▶ **Getting Around Town Safely.**
- **Identify your taxicab.** When riding in a taxicab alone or late at night, use a cellular phone to call a friend or pretend you are calling someone. Mention the cab number and your expected time of arrival. The driver now thinks that someone is expecting his cab to show up at the hotel at a specific time.

- **Carry hotel matchbooks, stationary, or postcards with the hotel name and address on it.** When the cab driver asks you where you want to go you don't have to say it out loud, just hand them the printed information. Not only is this safer, it gets you to the right place.

  I still remember the time I was in New York City as a media spokesperson. I was given a driver and a full schedule of magazine editors to visit including an afternoon appointment with Fit Magazine at 419 Park Ave South. We arrived right on schedule, but it didn't take long to find out that I was at 419 Park Ave – not 419 Park Ave *South*. By the time the driver drove me to the correct address, I was 15 minutes late! He later shared that he was hard of hearing! Needless to say, I always put my destination on paper now.

- **Have a native business contact escort you around.** Kroll Associates security firm rates Mexico City as the most dangerous city in the world and suggests sticking with hotel-ordered sedans rather than the more common VW bug taxis.

- **Be alert in crowded places.** Any crowded place is prime for thieves. Peak pick-pocketing activity is during the morning and evening rush hours on public transportation and walkways. Don't make it easy for the thieves, stay alert and keep your wallet and bags in your control.

▶ **Protect Your Belongings.**

- **Rip off old destination tags** before you check-in. If the ticket agent doesn't see them, your bag could get sent to the wrong city.

- **Leave identification on the inside of your luggage.** Don't rely just on the name tag on the outside, it can easily get ripped off. It's always a good idea to place a copy of your itinerary (including your destination hotel) and contact information inside the suitcase.

155

- **Tuck business cards into your jacket, coat, and brief-case.** In case you accidentally leave them behind in a restaurant or a bus or train, they'll know who to contact.

- **Tape a business card to the bottom of your laptop.** Thieves often don't look there and this often helps in identifying items when they're found.

- **Lock your luggage.** Although most luggage locks are not heavy-duty, they help to keep out curious fingers. Plastic cable ties (found in the hardware store) work just as well. Just don't forget to pack a knife or scissors to cut them. If your bag is well-worn, consider taping it shut or wrapping it in an orange garbage bag. These techniques make your bags safer from pilfering and easy to spot.

- **Don't check your luggage.** If your trip would be a disaster if your luggage got lost, consider not checking it. You can pack for a week in just one bag if you learn how to travel light. Carry-on luggage also saves time at your destination – you don't have to wait at baggage and you beat the long lines at the rental car or taxi line.

- **Keep valuable documents and belongings on your body.** Place your passport, credit cards, bank cards, plane tickets, traveler's checks, and large bills in a money belt, neck pouch, waist wallet, or in your clothing's secret pockets. Keep your passport, ticket, and photo ID readily available for check-in and customs. This will prevent you from needing to open your bag for everyone to see what you have in it.

- **Use a small fanny pack or purse for nonessentials**. This includes maps, lipstick, sunglasses, and a small amount of local currency. Purses should have a wide shoulder strap and be worn across your body with the purse in the front center of your body. To prevent a strap from getting sliced, invest in a chain-reinforced purse or fanny pack. Always give up your purse if someone tries to mug you.

- **Put your wallet in your front pocket.** It's just too easy to pickpocket your wallet from the back pocket. Use your front trouser pockets and wrap your wallet with several rubber bands in both directions to make it harder to remove. Several travel companies offer travel pants with zippers in the pockets.
- **Trick the thieves.** Use the local grocery plastic bag to carry your camera, maps, and other possessions that identify you as a tourist. Keep valuables in unexpected places such as film containers or in the toes of your stinky sneakers back in the hotel.

▶ **Watch Your Bags Closely.** Others may be watching it also!

- **Make your luggage distinguishable** so you can find it easily and no one accidentally or purposely takes yours. If you already have black luggage like everyone else, make yours stand out with bright stickers or a colorful luggage strap or luggage tag. You'll find a wide assortment at www.travelaccessories.com.
- **Don't lose sight of your bags.** When getting into the shuttle or taxi, make sure all your luggage is onboard before getting in yourself. Once our taxi driver left one piece of our luggage on the airport curb. We were lucky to have found it at the Airport Security an hour later. Often there is so much commotion at the airport, it's easy for a piece of luggage to get lifted. If you entrust a porter or are checking in at the airline ticket counter, keep your luggage in front of you and then don't leave until you see your luggage go down the conveyor belt.
- **Don't hang your handbag or carry-on over hooks in bathroom stalls.** Place your bags between your legs on clean paper. Or select an end stall where there are fewer angles to grab from.
- **Stow your carry-on** *across* **the airplane aisle from your seat** (instead of directly overhead) so you can keep an eye on them. Put them a few rows ahead of you.

157

How to Stay Healthy & Fit on the Road

- **Go directly to the luggage carousel.** Sure you're hungry, but most airports don't have security to protect anyone else from taking your bags. So go directly to baggage. If the bags are not up yet, you may want to rent your car or make a phone call as long as you can watch the carousel.
- **Hold onto your luggage.** Place your luggage directly in front of you (or between your feet) so you can see it at all times. Wrap a strap around your leg when making a phone call, checking email, or eating at the airport. As tempting as it may be, don't ask strangers to watch your bags while you use the rest room. They may not watch it carefully.
- **Keep your carry-on and briefcase with you** instead of leaving them unattended in the luggage room, trucker's lounges, or airline club's cloak room.

▶ Use ATM Machines Wisely.
- **Use only ATMs in well-lit, open areas.** Lock the car doors and roll up the other windows when you use a drive-through ATM. When using an indoor ATM that requires your card to open the door, close the door behind you so strangers can't come in with you. Do not leave your keys or valuables in the car when stepping out to use an ATM – even if no one is around.
- **Have your ATM card ready.** You don't want to be distracted by having to go through your wallet or purse.
- **Use your body and hands to hide your PIN** and transaction amount.
- **Don't count your cash** while standing at the ATM – put your cash, card, and receipt away immediately.
- **Cancel your transaction and leave immediately if you see anything suspicious.** As soon as possible confirm with your financial institution that the transaction was canceled.

▶ **Keep Records.**

- **Leave a copy of your itinerary back home.** In addition to the copy you keep in your checked luggage, give a contact person back home your itinerary and a copy of your passport information page in the event that you are delayed or don't show up as planned.

- **Make a record of your belongings**. Take photos of your luggage and valuable contents. Write down serial numbers of computers, cameras, and other valuable electronics for quick identification should something get stolen.

- **Record the numbers** of credit cards, traveler's checks (serial numbers and denomination), and ATM bank cards. Write down the 800 numbers in the event they are lost or stolen and you need to call them. And report the loss to the local police as well. Leave a copy with someone at home and keep one in your personal safe-keeping in a place separate from your money.

- **Take all receipts.** Don't leave ATM and credit card receipts behind which contain your numbers.

▶ **Drive Safely**

- **Avoid using the cell phone while driving**. A recent 1997 study published in the New England Journal of Medicine reports that "people who use cell phones while driving are four times more likely to be involved in traffic crashes as non-users." Some US cities and many entire countries have banned the use of cell phones while driving. Others prohibit using a cell phone without the use of a hand free device. So pull over!

- **Get out of their blind spots**. Your 3000 pound car doesn't stand a chance in a collision with an 80,000 pound truck. Stay out of their blind spots – directly behind, in front of, and on both sides of the truck.

- **Don't take it out on the road.** Don't express your anger and frustration to other drivers on the road. It helps to give yourself plenty of time, identify alternate routes, and relax with your favorite listening music.

How to Stay Healthy & Fit on the Road

- **Avoid aggressive drivers** who exceed the speed limit, follow too closely, make hand or facial gestures, or don't follow traffic rules. Make sure you're not contributing to the problem such as not giving others adequate space to merge or driving slowly in the left lane. When you encounter an angry driver, pull back and give them plenty of space, avoid eye contact, and don't challenge their behavior. If you believe the driver is following you or trying to start a fight, drive to a place where other people are around such as a police station, hospital, or shopping center. Do not get out of your car (blow the horn for help) and do not go immediately home.

- **Take a nap if you're tired.** According to the National Sleep Foundation (NSF) survey about half of adults in the US said they drove while drowsy in the past year; nearly one out of five (17%) have actually dozed off while driving. While a good night's sleep may be the best solution to prevent this deadly fatigue, a quick power nap (10-20 minutes) provides some short term alertness when you're feeling drowsy. Caffeine, the equivalence of two cups of coffee, can also provide some short term relief from sleepiness, but may also add to insomnia later in the day. The effectiveness of opening the window or listening to the radio has not been demonstrated. If you're going to stop for a snack, walk, or nap, be sure to pull off onto a safe exit. If you power nap in your car, it's best to pull into a busy truck stop or restaurant in a well-lighted area.

▶ **Traveling Alone? Don't Stand Out.** Single travelers are more susceptible to crime so, when at all possible, don't let people know that you're traveling by yourself.

- **Ask for two keys**. Make your hotel reservations as if you're married and always request two keys at the hotel registration desk. Even if you're not concerned that someone is watching you, it's always better to have two. There's always a chance that one of the keys won't work or that you'll leave one of the keys in the room when you step out.

- **Order room service for two.** Do you ever order breakfast the evening before by specifying what you want and hanging the order on the outside doorknob? Instead of announcing to everyone passing down the hall that you're traveling alone, either call in the order or ask for two place settings. Another option is to ask for two cups with the carafe of coffee.

- **Don't look like you're alone.** When strolling the streets, walk with a group. If it's late and you're alone, ask someone from the front desk to accompany you to your room or to your car. If your room is on the lower hotel floor, consider keeping the curtains closed.

Traveling Outside the Country

A visit to a foreign country need not be any more worrisome than visiting another city in the United States if you consider the following:

▶ **Check with the State Department.** Did you know that it is illegal to bring chewing gum into Singapore? Use of hand-held cellular phones while driving in Hong Kong is prohibited? And that people bringing prescription drugs into Zambia without a physician's prescription may be arrested and incarcerated? Prior to travel outside of the United States, log onto www.state.gov/travel to find valuable information including:

- **Travel warnings and consular information sheets.** Here you'll find: country description, crime information, traffic safety and road conditions, aviation safety oversight information, criminal penalties, and more - for 200+ countries. This information may also be obtained from any regional passport agency, most airline computer reservation systems, or by calling the Bureau of Consular Affairs at (202) 647-5225. You can also dial 202-647-3000 from your fax machine and follow the prompts to receive information.

- **Background Notes.** This section includes information about the country's geography and weather, its people

161

(including languages, religion, education, health), the government and principal government officials, economy (GDP, unemployment rate, major products and agriculture, natural resources, and history), history of the country and its people, foreign relations, and the current political situation. Copies can also be purchased from Superintendent of Documents (202-512-1800).

- **US Embassies and Consulates information.** Includes names of key officers, address, and telephone and fax numbers. Also identifies emergency and non-emergency services that consulate officers can provide to American citizens. (http://usembassy.state.gov)

- **Foreign entry requirements.** While your passport shows proof of citizenship, a visa or tourist card grants you permission to visit that country for a specified purpose and a limited time. Information for both are available on this site (or go directly to www.travel.state.gov/passport_services.html) including passport application forms. Or call the Passport Information Center at 1-900-225-5674 or 1-888-362-8668 with a credit card.

- **Lists of doctors, hospitals, and lawyers abroad**

- **Customs regulations.** This includes required duty, Internal Revenue tax, and exemptions for items purchased outside the country.

- **Tips for travelers.** This area of the web site covers currency, dual nationality, import and export controls, restrictions on use of photography, and warnings on the use of drugs. You'll also find helpful precautions to minimize the chance of becoming a victim of crime or terrorism.

▶ **Protect Your Passport.** Your passport confirms your citizenship so guard it carefully. You will need it, not just for travel, but also when you pick up mail or check into hotels, embassies or consulates.

- **Do not use it as collateral** for a loan or lend it to anyone.

- **You may be required to leave it overnight.** When entering some countries or registering at hotels, you may be asked to fill out a police card listing your name, passport number, destination, local address, and your reason for travel. You may be required to leave your passport at the hotel reception desk overnight so that it can be checked by local police officials. This is a normal procedure required by local laws. If your passport is not returned the following morning, immediately report the impoundment to local police authorities and to the nearest US embassy or consulate.

- **Hide it securely on your person.** Do not place it in your luggage, in a handbag, or in an exposed pocket. Whenever possible leave your passport in the hotel safe, not in an empty hotel room. One family member should not carry all the passports for the entire family.

- **Carry extra pictures of yourself.** When traveling internationally, take a photocopy of your actual passport, plus additional passport photos and proof of citizenship. Pack them separately from your original passport. If you were to lose the original, you will encounter fewer challenges in obtaining a new passport from the American Embassy. The extra pictures may also come in handy for bus passes or other local passes.

▶ **Bring Adequate Money.** It is wise to carry most of your money in traveler's checks and not carry large amounts of cash.

- **Exchange some of your money before you leave.** It's helpful to have a small amount of foreign currency for buses, taxis, phones, or tips prior to boarding the plane since banks and foreign exchange facilities may not be open when you arrive.

- **Check with your credit card company.** Call to see if your credit cards can be used worldwide and be replaced if it's stolen internationally. Keep track of your credit card purchases so that you do not exceed your limit. Travelers have been arrested overseas for mistakenly

163

exceeding their credit limit! Bringing one or two credit cards is adequate – leave the others at home.

- **Have enough money to pay an airport departure tax when you leave the country.** Check with the airline or travel agent; it can be as high as $50.

▶ **Prepare for Emergency Funds.**

- **Check with your ATM service.** Before leaving on your trip, check with your bank to see if the country or countries that you plan to visit have Automated Teller Machine (ATM) service that you can use with your card. You'll find listings at www.mastercard.com and www.visa.com.

- **Take your bank's telephone number.** This will come in handy if you run out of cash and need to transfer money. In some countries, major banks and certain travel agencies can help arrange a transfer of funds from your account to a foreign bank.

- **Make arrangements with a relative or friend.** If you do not have a bank account from which you can obtain emergency funds, make arrangements in advance with a relative or friend to send you emergency funds should it become necessary. The US Embassy or consulate can help you arrange a money wire transfer if you find yourself in a jam.

▶ **Check into Driving Requirements.**

- **Obtain an international driver's permit.** If the country you are visiting does not recognize a US driver's license, you'll need to obtain an international driver's permit. The US Department of State has authorized two organizations to issue international driving permits to those who hold valid US driver's licenses: AAA (www.aaa.com) and the American Automobile Touring Alliance (www.nationalautoclub.com, 650-294-7000)

- **Get a road permit.** Certain countries require road permits, instead of tolls, to use on their divided highways, and they will fine those found driving without a permit.

- **Consider additional auto insurance.** Car rental agencies overseas usually provide auto insurance but in some countries the required coverage is minimal. When renting a car overseas, consider purchasing insurance coverage that is at least equivalent to that which you carry at home. In general, your US auto insurance may cover you in Canada and Mexico but may not cover you when driving in other countries. Even if your policy is valid in one of these countries, it may not meet its minimum requirements. If you are under-insured for a country, auto insurance can usually be purchased on either side of the border.

▶ **Consider Travel Insurance.** Depending on the plan, travel insurance usually promises to cover you for cancellation or interruption of your trip, some form of emergency medical care while you are traveling, lost or stolen luggage, and various other troublesome occurrences.

- **Investigate your current coverage.** You may not need travel insurance if you are already adequately covered by other insurance policies. Your homeowners or tenants insurance may cover the loss or theft of your luggage. Certain credit cards may provide travel insurance if you have used them to purchase the ticket for your trip. Check any other agreements you have with your travel agent, tour operator, airline, or other companies involved with your travel plans. If you have a fully refundable airline ticket, you may not need trip cancellation/interruption insurance.
- **Read the fine print.** Before you decide on a travel insurance plan, it is wise to investigate the plan carefully and read the fine print. Do they cover the financial costs in case of situations including a sudden, serious injury or illness to you, a family member, or a traveling companion? Will they reimburse you if there is a financial default of the airline, cruise line or tour operator? Do they cover natural disasters or strikes that impede travel

165

services or a terrorist incident? How about if you, a traveling member of your family, or a traveling companion were quarantined, served with a court order or required to serve on a jury; or a circumstance in which you were directly involved in an accident enroute to departure for your trip?

▶ **Beware of the Following Purchases.** It is important that you keep all receipts for items you buy overseas. They will be helpful in making your US Customs declaration when you return. Be cautious about these items:

- **Fresh fruit, meat, vegetables, plants in soil, and many other agricultural products from abroad.** These are prohibited entry into the United States (and sometimes from state to state) because they may carry foreign insects and diseases that could damage US crops, forests, gardens, and livestock. These rules also apply to mailed products from overseas. Prohibited items will be confiscated and destroyed. For more information log onto www.usda.gov.

- **Some wildlife souvenirs.** Live, wild animals or articles made from animals and plants cannot be brought legally into the US. In addition to being confiscated by government inspectors, you could face other penalties for attempting to bring them in. More information is available at www.worldwide.org or by calling 202-293-4800.

- **Glazed ceramic ware.** While it is legal to bring into the country, you can suffer lead poisoning if you consume food or beverages that are stored or served in improperly glazed ceramics. The US Food and Drug Administration recommends that ceramic tableware purchased abroad be tested for lead release by a commercial laboratory on your return or be used for decorative purposes only. More information is available at www.fda.gov or by calling 1-800-532-4440.

- **Antiques.** Certain countries consider antiques to be national treasures and the "inalienable property of the nation." In some countries, customs authorities seize illegally purchased antiques without compensation and they may also levy fines on the purchaser. Americans have been arrested and prosecuted for purchasing antiques without a permit or for purchasing reproductions of antiques from street vendors if a local authority believed the purchase was a national treasure. Document your purchases as authentic or reproductions and secure the necessary export permit through the country's national museum or a reputable dealer. If you have questions about purchasing antiques, the country's tourist office can guide you. If you still have doubts, consult the Consular Section of the nearest US embassy or consulate.

▶ **Get the Paperwork Ready for Immigration and Customs.** Items may include: passport, International Certificate of Vaccination, a medical letter, and Customs certificate of registration for foreign-made personal articles (discussed below). When returning to the United States by car from Mexico or Canada, have your certificate of vehicle registration available.

• **Pre-register with US Customs.** Foreign-made personal articles (such as watches, cameras, and video recorders) taken abroad are subject to US Customs duty and tax upon your return unless you have proof of prior possession such as a receipt, bill of sale, an insurance policy, or a jeweler's appraisal. If you do not have proof of prior possession, that can be identified by serial number or permanent markings, you may take them to the Customs office nearest you, or to the port of departure for registration, *before* you depart the US. The certificate of registration will expedite free entry of these items when you return home.

▶ **Obey Foreign Laws.** When you are in a foreign country, you are subject to its laws. It helps to learn about local laws and regulations avoid areas of unrest and disturbance.

- **Deal only with authorized outlets** when exchanging money or buying airline tickets and traveler's checks.

- **Do *not* deliver a package for anyone.** You've heard that foreign laws overseas are more severe than US laws when it comes to buying or selling drugs. So don't deliver a package for anyone unless you know the person well and you are certain that the package does not contain drugs or other contraband.

- **Learn about local regulations before selling personal effects**, such as clothing, cameras, or jewelry; the penalties may be severe.

- **Think before you snap.** Since some countries are sensitive about what you can photograph, check with the country's tourist office or its embassy or consulate in the US. In general, refrain from photographing police and military installations and personnel; industrial structures, including harbor, rail, and airport facilities; border areas; and scenes of civil disorder or other public disturbance. Taking such photographs may result in your detention, in the confiscation of your camera and films, as well as the imposition of fines.

Medical Safety

When you're planning to travel abroad, consider these:

▶ **Get Adequate Health Insurance.** Obtaining medical treatment and hospital care can be costly for travelers who are injured or who become seriously ill overseas.

- **Your Health Insurance Provider.** Although many (not all) health insurance companies will pay "customary and reasonable" hospital costs abroad, very few will pay for medical evacuation back to the United States.

- **Get supplemental insurance.** For that reason, The Department of State (202-647-3000, www.state.gov) suggests you consider purchasing supplemental insurance to cover the very costly medical evacuation. Medpass is a for-profit company that arranges for air and surface evacuation back to United States. For details, call 800-860-1111.

- **The Social Security Medicare/Medicaid program** does *not* provide coverage for hospital or medical services outside the United States. Senior citizens may wish to contact the American Association of Retired Persons (AARP) for information about foreign medical care coverage with Medicare supplement plans.

▶ **Visit with a Travel Medicine Doctor.** See your doctor at least 4-6 weeks before your planned travel to get information on immunization, health records, and testing requirements (such as HIV testing).

- **Find a specialist.** Your physician can give you a referral locally. To find one when you're traveling, contact The American Society of Tropical Medicine and Hygiene (847-480-9592, www.astmh.org) or the Department of State Bureau of Consular Affair (www.state.gov/travel or autofax service at 202-647-3000).

- **Get a tetanus shot** if it's been 10 years since your last one.

- **Get your flu shot.** A flu vaccine will offer protection for just 4 months. In the states, flu shots are given towards the end of the year. If you're planning a trip to the southern hemisphere during their peak flu season (April-September), ask your doctor about another flu shot.

- **Get the necessary immunizations.** If vaccinations are required, they must be recorded on approved forms often available through your doctor or public health office.

- **Check with the CDC.** Six weeks prior to your departure oversees contact the Center for Disease Control for country-specific information (www.cdc.gov/travel, 877-FYI-TRIP, 877-394-8747). You'll find out about health advisories and outbreaks, immunization recommendations or requirements, advice on food and drinking water safety, and tips for special needs travelers.

How to Stay Healthy & Fit on the Road

▶ **Bring Necessary Medical Documentation**

- **Health and insurance information**. Note your allergies, diseases, or conditions on a piece of paper in your purse or wallet, detailing what to do, and emergency contact information. Write this in English and in the languages of the countries you will be visiting. For serious conditions, wear a medical bracelet as well.

- **Health insurance information**. If your policy covers medical expenses outside of the country, carry both your insurance policy card and a claim form.

- **A letter from your doctor.** If you go abroad with pre-existing medical problems, carry a letter from you doctor describing your condition, including information on your prescription medicines (and their generic names).

- **Keep prescriptions in their original, labeled containers.** Although it's tempting to consolidate all your pills, leave medicines in their original, labeled containers for ease in customs processing.

- **Consult the embassy or consulate.** Before you leave the US, contact the embassy or consulate (www.state.gov/travel) of those countries you'll be visiting for precise information. A doctor's certificate may not suffice as authorization to transport all prescription drugs to foreign countries. Travelers have innocently been arrested for drug violations when carrying items not considered as narcotics in the United States.

Have a safe trip!

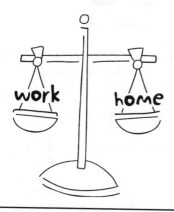

Chapter 8

Staying Balanced

In This Chapter:
▶Maintaining the Home Front
▶Staying Connected on the Road
▶Enjoying Your Time Off
▶Blending Work and Family

Time is not elastic, you can't stretch it. Each of us are given just 168 hours in a week, no more, no less. In the *Putting the Brakes on Stress* chapter, you were asked to consider what your lifelong priorities are. To have the time to do what's really important to you, you'll need to streamline (or even eliminate) those things of lesser importance. The following tips suggestions will help you successfully balance your home and work life.

Maintaining the Home Front

Everyone at one time or another has found it difficult to balance life. Travelers find it even more challenging. When home seems more like work than a refuge from work, it's time to initiate a change. Admit that you don't have time to do everything and taking care of the house and yard is not your number one priority when you're home. If you want to make the home more peaceful, here are some ideas that have worked for road warriors:

▶ **Get Rid of the Clutter.** While too much gunk on your car's spark plugs can cause misfiring, too much junk in your house can cause misdirection of your priorities.

- **Do a spring cleaning.** Go through your stuff and trash what you don't need including clothes you haven't worn in a year.

- **Keep the clutter from coming back.** Make a new rule that every time you buy something, you'll throw something else away.

- **Stop subscriptions** to nonessential magazines, newsletters, and newspapers if you don't have time to read them. Seeing the stacks pile up only adds to your guilt and stress.

▶ **Get Organized.** To reduce stress and save time looking for things, organize your house so there's a place for everything. In addition:

- **Shop in bulk.** It saves time and money. Shop for paper goods, bathroom products, and cleaning supplies in huge quantities every few months so you're never running to the store for just one thing.

- **Always have a back up.** Get everyone in the household involved in keeping a running shopping list on a notepad (perhaps posted on the refrigerator). When you open the bottle of your favorite salad dressing, jot it down on the list. Don't wait until the bottle is empty.

- **Find a grocery store that delivers.** See if there's an online grocery delivery service in your area or a local grocery store that will accept a faxed order and have it ready for pick up on your way into town.

- **Put it in a place that makes sense**. Pat Moore, the Queen of Clutter and author of *Tip A Day To Keep Your Clutter at Bay*, suggests setting up a correspondence center. Drop your mail here and have all the supplies you need to pay the bills: checks, stamps, return address labels, calculator, and pen.

- **Have a written schedule.** Set routines that the family can easily follow, decide who's in charge of what, and when they need to do it. Then post the schedule in a conspicuous place so there are no misunderstandings.
- **Keep a family master calendar.** To keep everyone in the family informed, keep one master calendar posted at home with everyone's activities (including your travel).

▶ **Lower Your Standards.** This is a hard one, especially if you're a perfectionist. But be honest with yourself. If you try to do every task perfectly, you won't have time to do all the things that are important to you. Don't lower your standards about everything, just the things that really don't matter in the long run. Remember the old saying: "If it's not life or limb, the heck with it."

- **Have a picnic.** Use paper plates and plastic ware to save on kitchen cleanup time.
- **Simplify the tasks.** Replace the bedspread with an easy-care comforter. The bed skirt always makes the bottom of the bed look neat. Tuck away some of those dust-collecting knickknacks. Are you still folding your underwear? Just because Mom used to do it, doesn't mean that you have to. Instead, just throw them in the drawer – the wrinkles will come out when you put them on. I promise! Simplify your bill paying by writing checks just once a month, using a check-writing system on your computer, or set up your bills for automatic payment. Each idea doesn't sound like much of a savings, but if you give yourself just one extra minute a day you'll have more than six hours throughout the year! What if you could save 10 minutes a day?
- **Stop feeling guilty.** Turn off the home and garden TV shows if they make you feel guilty about not having a picture perfect home. A woman in one of my seminars told me that she always keeps the vacuum cleaner in her living room. If anyone drops by, she would ease her guilt of a less than perfect home by telling them "I was

just getting started on my cleaning." Our parents had to rid themselves of the guilt of not ironing the bed sheets, it's time for you to realize that "good enough" is enough for a lot of things around the house.

- **Simplify the yard work.** If you don't find yard and garden work relaxing, it may be time to replace some of the gardens with an easy-care lawn, remind yourself that the fallen leaves make good fertilizer, or move into a condo where someone else does it for you.

- **Do it less often.** Sure it's nice to have the bathroom cleaned every day, but will once a week suffice? Can you change the bed sheets less often?

▶ **Ask for Help Around the House.** Chances are, there are people around who are willing to help out if you just ask.

- **Hand over some of the responsibilities to your spouse and kids.** It's true, they won't complete the task the same way you do, but does it really matter? Although it's OK to instruct them generally how to do a task, consider their age and experience. If you continually comment about the way they complete the work, you'll only add to the stress. And if you redo their work, you've let them off the hook (which may be just what they intended). Be patient and give it time. When I first began to travel, my daughter was just four. During my five and six day trips, she began helping out by unloading the dishwasher with her dad. Now she cleans up the whole kitchen, pitches in with yard work, and makes dinner.

- **Get a service contract.** What can you give up in order to fit a yard, pool, or house cleaning service into your budget? In the Houston summers, when I was gone more than five days, it would cost me $25 to treat the algae build up in my pool. Since a pool service company supplied the chemicals, I found it less expensive to have a pool service. For shear luxury, have the house cleaning service come just before you arrive home so you can just come home and enjoy it.

- **Ask a friend or neighbor.** Look around. Is there a friend or neighbor (even a kid) who you can trust to come by regularly to water plants, feed animals, and pick up mail? Even if you don't need things done on a regular basis, give them a house key for urgent matters. Instead of paying them, you may consider using your frequent flier miles and inviting them on your next business trip to someplace fun.

- **Take advantage of Mom.** Some travelers, who have long left the nest, commented that they have taken advantage of their (often divorced or widowed) mother. If they have the time, mothers often enjoy cooking, sharing news, and running errands.

▶ **Get Help with the Kids.** Are you the main caretaker? Then:

- **Arrange a car pool.** Instead of trying to do it all, arrange a car pool with other parents who take kids to the same school or event. Chances are, they'll be grateful that you asked. Keep a list of car pool phone numbers with you at all times for emergencies.

- **Keep kids occupied with after school activities.** Instead of different plans for each day, make it easy on yourself. Find one program that is right in the school or has a bus that picks them up from school.

- **Find a "rent-a-mom"** to pick up kids after school, take them to the after school events, and who does light housekeeping and laundry.

▶ **Set Limits on your Commitments.** Besides work and family, what other obligations do you have? You may need to:

- **Cut back on volunteer hours.** Sure, giving back to society is a good thing to do and it's even stress-relieving (in the right amount), but do you have to sign up for everything? If you're not fulfilling your major priorities, it's time to say no.

175

- **Narrow down family activities and obligations.** Whether it's the kid's activities or your extended family obligations, you might find yourself at an event every day of every weekend. Ask your spouse and kids; you might find that they too need a break.

Staying Connected on the Road

Have you ever returned from a trip and felt like a stranger in your own home? You can avoid this by being in their hearts and minds even when you're physically not there. The following suggestions will help to bridge distances between you and those you care about.

▶ **Bring Reminders from Home.**
- **Pack a family picture.** Bring a framed picture, laminate a picture to use as a bookmark, or pack a small "talking picture frame" that allows your loved ones to record a short message for you to play over and over (www.Brookstone.com has one set in an alarm clock).
- **Take a copy of the family schedule.** Instead of simply asking them how their day was, ask them a specific question about one of their activities that day.
- **Make copies of your kid's homework.** My daughter likes it when I can give her a spelling test, help with her math problems, or help her study for the science test. Find out how to best keep in touch with the coaches and teachers. Email might be easier than calling.
- **Put your loved ones in your planner.** Keep addresses and phone numbers of family and friends that you want to keep in touch with. Set alarms for birthdays, anniversaries, and other special days that you want to remember to call or write.

▶ **Leave Some Love Behind.** While others understand, the little ones really miss you when you're gone.

- **Keep them involved.** Put your trip down on the calendar including how to reach you, where you'll be (perhaps with pictures), and with a big smiley face when you'll be returning.

- **Leave love notes behind.** Before you leave, write short notes for everyday that you're away. Have someone give them to your children at breakfast or put them in their lunchbox. Or leave the love notes yourself in their clothing, bathroom drawers, under the pillow, in the dryer, or inside the refrigerator. Whether an elaborate game or a simple process, it will always be meaningful.

- **Tape your messages before you leave.** Think up messages for your loved ones and either audio or video tape them ahead of time or record it on the road. You could tape one for each day that you're on the road to remind them of what they need to bring to school, that it's trash day, and that you love them. They will treasure these for the rest of their lives.

- **Keep up some of the usual activities.** If you're the main cook, before you leave town, you may want to plan some simple menus and do the shopping. Or make a large meal so there's plenty to eat – including leftovers.

- **Treat them to dinner.** Show them you care, by giving them a few gift certificates for their favorite restaurants – this makes it an easy decision to go out to eat while you're away.

- **Plan the kid's clothing.** For the little ones, bundle their daily clothes (tops, bottoms, socks, underwear, and accessories) with a band. Tuck a little note or picture in each.

177

▶ **Stay in Touch.**

- **Surprise them with a call.** Even if you call every night at a designated time, make other calls as a surprise – when you are free to listen to their day. Perhaps a good morning call, when kids come home from school, or during your spouse's lunch break.

- **Give them a journal.** Sometimes at the end of the day, they're too tired to remember what happened. Give them their personal notebook or journal so they can jot down a few notes throughout the day to jog their memory when you call.

- **Tell them about your day.** Communicate about everything so they feel they are part of your life on the road. Tell them about the funny and not-so-funny events. Keep a running list of things you need to talk with them about – a weird thing that happened, their homework, or a news event.

- **Keep them informed.** People worry about you when you travel. So ease their mind with an "I love you call" when you make it to the airport or hotel. And call just as soon as you land back in your hometown.

- **Go cordless.** Consider a cordless phone at home so your family can talk when they're getting the mail, cooking dinner, or checking on the kids. This makes you feel more like you're there and makes it easier for them to continue with their routine at home.

- **Get personal 800 numbers.** Set up one that rings at home so you can call without having to pay calling card surcharges or worry about your calling card number getting stolen at the airport. An 800 number also simplifies things when you need to call from other people's offices. You can also use a personal 800 number to be forwarded to your hotel so friends and family can always be in touch without having your itinerary.

- **Find an inexpensive way to keep in touch** so it doesn't become a financial burden. Check out the different calling cards or buy more minutes on your cellular phone. If time zones and work schedules make it difficult to talk directly, consider a voice pager where you and they can leave messages. Don't forget to use a phone service or credit card that gives you airline miles so you can earn more free travel for your family.

- **Be accessible.** Get a beeper or mobile phone that only your family and friends have the phone number to. It gives you a peace of mind knowing that they can always get in touch with you and makes them feel like you're not so far away. These calls tend to be more spontaneous. You can always turn it off or use the caller-ID when you're in an important meeting. If you don't want to buy one, consider renting one from the rental car companies.

- **Read to your children.** Carry on the bedtime routine by bringing a book you can read to them over the phone. Or audiotape a story to give to them before you leave.

- **Start your own version of the "Never Ending Story."** This can address the fact (and fiction) associated with Mom/Dad on the road. They'll look forward to those stories for years on end.

- **Install web cameras on your laptop and home computers.** Now they can show you their artwork, grades, or new haircut. Or take the digital video camera with you to tape your travels (even your hotel room) to show them back home.

▶ **Send Them Reminders That You're Thinking of Them.**

- **Order flowers** to be sent home on special occasions when you can't be there.

- **Drop a postcard in the mail.** Share a few historical facts, interesting things about the city, or tell them about something funny that happened on your trip. Take advantage of the free postcards in the hotel or send the tacky tourist postcards! With so much electronic media, we forget the power of a handwritten note.

- **Tape your own messages on the road.** Instead of writing or calling, use a mini recorder to tape letters to friends and family. On extended trips, invite them to do

179

the same back to you. It's personal and is effective when time zone differences make it difficult to connect.

- **Keep note cards and stamped envelopes with you.** It's easy to keep in touch if you have pre-addressed, pre-stamped envelopes.

- **Email your family.** Some children and teenagers are more likely to open up in email rather than on the phone. Send an instant message if they're on-line and you can't get through on the phone. If you have a digital camera you can transmit instant postcards home.

- **Fax it.** With so many home offices, many of us have a fax at home. Why don't you fax them a note? My daughter and I exchange hand-drawn artwork on a regular basis.

- **Send form letters.** You know those form letters you get at Christmas time? Why not send friends and extended family a form letter every now and then to let them know you're thinking of them. Don't forget a hand-written personal note at the bottom.

▶ **Bring Back a Gift.** While some travelers bring home a gift on every trip, others make it more special by finding something really unique every once in awhile. Then again, you may want to consider giving them a gift *before* you leave town or dropping one in the mail while you're away. It can be fun to scout the new city for that special gift; other times it's easier to pack a gift from home just in case you don't have time to shop. Here are some gift ideas:

- **Something from the room.** Little kids are impressed by small things that travelers take for granted, such as hotel chocolates or candies, small bottles of shampoo or lotion, or the miniature bottle of ketchup from room service.

- **Something from the conventions.** Wouldn't sponsoring companies be mortified to find out how much of their tradeshow giveaways are enjoyed by our kids? Our kids love the personalized sunglasses, key chains, pens and pencils, pocket knives, key chains, tote bags, umbrellas, coffee mugs, rulers, and all the other freebies.

- **Something snuggly.** Who doesn't like a stuffed animal?

- **Something local.** Get something that the city, state, or country you're visiting is famous for. Perhaps a postcard with local information, a rock, T-shirt, or coffee mug. It could be San Francisco's sourdough bread, a miniature Eiffel Tower keyring, or a Portuguese fisherman sweater.

- **Something small.** Gifts don't have to be big or expensive. Consider bringing home small shadow miniatures to collect, bean bag animals, or magic tricks.

- **Something goofy.** Hotel gift shops are often full of funny refrigerator magnets and toys poking fun of the local area.

- **Something sporty.** If the kids (or your spouse) is into sports, bring home a momento of the local team.

Enjoying Your Time Off

Do you ever find yourself thinking about home when you're at work or worrying about your job when you're with friends and family? Here are some thoughts on how to stay on track:

▶**Compartmentalize.** Ideally, you want to "stay in the present" by giving 100% while you're at work and then be able to be there 100% for your family and friends during your off hours. How can we achieve this disciplined focus?

- **Plan your day.** Remember that it will never all be done. So prioritize what needs to get done, know your limitations, and pace yourself accordingly. Stop comparing yourself to other people. Chances are they're not as perfect as they appear either.

- **Jot down notes.** Stay in the present by giving all your attention to what you are working on now. If you're with family or friends and your mind drifts to work-related tasks or problems, take a moment to jot yourself a note of what needs to be done or the questions you have. Writing down those thoughts helps to remove them as

181

distractions. When your mind begins to wander again, and it will, remind yourself that they're written down so you don't have to continue thinking about them. Then, schedule a time later on in the day or week to work on those issues.

- **Use on/off reminders.** It's important that you find cut-off reminders that work for you and then stick with them. For example, tell yourself that you will only think about work on these certain days and during these specific times. Make them realistic enough that you can keep your promise. Drivers coming home from visiting with a client may allow themselves to think about work until they leave the parking lot or hit a specific exit on the freeway. Or allow yourself to finish the report on the return flight; then direct your thoughts to personal issues on the drive home from the airport. One client told me that, on the way out of the office, he would imagine putting his work-related problems on the trees lining the walkway to the parking lot. Then he would forget about them. On the way back into work the next day, he would "pick them up" off the trees and direct his concentration back on work. These ideas may sound strange, but they really do work. Give it a try!

- **Hide your work.** Out of sight, out of mind really does work. If you find it difficult to forget work at the end of the day, hide any reminders in a separate room, box, or corner – and don't look at it! And, never take work to bed, especially if you have trouble sleeping.

- **Find balance.** Some travelers, instead of compartmentalizing work and home life, look for where personal and business goals blend and benefit each other. Some have formed a business with their spouse so they can work and play together. Others take their children on business trips.

▶ **Stay Tuned to the Right Station.** When you catch yourself worrying about things you can't control, things that don't matter long term, or things already on your priority list for another time, it's time to change stations.

- **Tell yourself to stop.** When your self-talk is getting the best of you, say to yourself: "Stop, stop, stop, stop."

- **Coach yourself.** If you've ever had a good coach, you recognize how important it is to stop dwelling on the downside and to think positive. Replace your negative thoughts with positive ones like "I can do it," "I feel good about this next opportunity," "I'm moving in the right direction," or "I'm working on that already." For example, instead of "I've been out all week; haven't made a single sale. I don't have what it takes. What if I lose my job?" Change your self-talk to: "This is a numbers game. Let's rethink what I'm saying. I need to tighten it up; things will change."

- **Stop "shoulding" on yourself.** When you berate yourself with comments like "I should have" or "I shouldn't have," recognize these comments as what they are – self-abuse. Instead, ask yourself what you'll do next time this happens. Replace that abusive, nonproductive talk with "Next time I will…" so you begin to turn mistakes into lessons learned.

- **Talk back to yourself.** When a worry pops into your mind, ask yourself if it really matters in the scheme of things. You might need to give yourself a pep talk. If there's a positive person in your life, think what they would say in this situation.

- **Don't forget to pack your sense of humor.** A healthy sense of humor will help you through missed or cancelled flights, lost luggage, and related hassles. In addition, pack extra patience, a pair of "perspective glasses" for looking at things from someone else's point of view, and a spare attitude when yours is destroyed by delays, late wakeup calls, and stains.

▶ **Schedule Time for Your Personal Life.** If business meetings are important enough for the day planner, so are your family and friends. So put them in your calendar along with your business meetings. If you don't, your personal life will keep coming in last. Few of us are really as critical to our business as we think we are. Remember that some amount of fun helps to keep us fresh in our work.

- **Treat Yourself Right.** If you pay attention, the flight attendant still does the routine about safety. He or she shows you how to use the oxygen mask and says "If you're traveling with someone, put your mask on first, then help others with theirs." The same rule applies with other things. It's important to take care of yourself first so you have the energy to help others. If you come home exhausted, you won't be any fun for your family.

- **Mark off critical days**. Cross off the dates that you want to stay at home (such as birthdays, anniversaries, and vacations) and keep them sacred. The more often you give in to work, the more likely they are to ask you again. So put your foot down about these important days!

- **Set limits at home.** Many of us find it easy to be lulled into working long hours when we're at home in the evenings and on off days. Set a limit of how much work you'll do when you're at home. This includes checking email and taking business related calls. You'll feel more refreshed if you keep at least one weekend day free even if it means working longer hours on workdays.

- **Deliberately schedule events during your off time.** It's great to relax on your weekends and be spontaneous with your time. But if you find it difficult to get away from work, plan your day. Include regular exercise or relaxation routines, hobbies, service organization or volunteer activities, social events, and family time. This will also prevent you from turning an off-day into an errand day. With less time available, you'll find more efficient ways of getting your errands done. I think it's healthy to spend the weekend outdoors at the park, the zoo, or on a hike. You can connect with your family a lot better without the TV and telephone and sunlight is helpful with jet lag as well.

- **Make a date with your spouse or partner**. "Dates" help to keep relationships strong and your personal life balanced. Think about a "date night" before you travel. And while on your trip, plan another date night for the first or second evening you get home to "debrief" about your time apart. A weekend get-a-way every few months can help to rekindle a relationship. Alternate who does the planning and try to be creative. Keep in mind that although you may be tired of eating out, your spouse may not have had the opportunity.

- **Be flexible.** When you return home (especially when you get an earlier flight), do something special like pick the kids up from school or surprise them at lunch. Work from home on travel days so you can have breakfast or lunch with your family, take kids to school, or something that you don't normally have time for.

- **Consider the best times to travel.** If you don't set some limits about when you'll travel, your work might continually cut into family and personal time. Have weekly family meetings to discuss upcoming travel and plan need-to-attend events such as ball games, ballet recitals, or the office picnic into your schedule as much as possible. Perhaps it's time to say no to weekend travel and take the first flight out on Monday. If you sleep well on planes, you may want to take the red-eye on Sunday night after you've tucked in the kids. While some travelers find it easier to be gone for just short trips, others like to bunch their needed travel together so they can allocate chunks for personal needs. Find out what works for you.

- **Schedule business travel close to the weekend.** On the other hand, regular travelers sometimes forget to take advantage of the perks that come with traveling. What you save by staying over on a Saturday often will pay for the extra days in the city. Check with the visitors bureau (the web sites are listed in chapter 9) to see

185

what's happening in the town. Perhaps you'll want to bring your spouse along, meet an old friend in the city, or treat yourself to that new museum exhibit you've been wanting to see.

▶ **Don't Feel Guilty about Travel.** My daughter was four when I took my speaking career outside of the Houston area and began to travel. I'll never forget that first phone call home. When I heard her crying hysterically about how she wished I was there, I questioned whether I had made the right choice. But things got better real fast and I began to realize that travel was not only good for me and my career, but it was enriching her life as well. They're better off – and so are you – when you travel some.

- **You can refocus.** Travelers, especially the primary care-takers in the family, often use this time away to rejuvenate their spirit and refocus their career.

- **Other relationships are built.** Remind yourself that your time away means bonding time with the other parent or caretaker. Alexandra cried less on each and every day. On day 5 she calmly told me about her day, said she missed me, and then said "I gotta go. Daddy and I are coloring." I found out, when I returned, that my husband had already begun to develop a different relationship than the one they had with me around. And over the years, it has continued to grow.

- **Your job teaches them about endless opportunities.** Traveling not only opens your eyes to more exciting and challenging options in life, it teaches your kids many things as well. I believe children become more open-minded, more positive about the world and its people, and gives them a love of travel.

- **They learn how to take care of themselves.** Without Mom around all the time, my husband and my daughter both took on more responsibilities. Alexandra not only learned how to pack her own lunch by first grade - she took pride in managing it herself. Lorin and Alexandra learned how to cooked dinner together. Their favorite meal, albeit simple, was more fun than any of my meals. It was a "face" of plain spaghetti noodles with eyes, nose, and mouth made of sausage - and broccoli hair. I've learned that Alexandra not only manages just fine without me around all the time, she's more confident and independent.

- **Your kids learn about the places you visit.** When you travel there are so many opportunities to teach your kids about the world. Keep a large map on a wall and put a colored pin into the city or cities you will be visiting. Bring back interesting brochures, magazines, and paper restaurant place mats which describe the local areas. Check the weather together (or ask them to do it if they're computer-savvy).

Blending Work and Family

I looked forward to the next trip just weeks after my first, yet I dreaded leaving Alexandra again for another six days. My concerns got more complicated when just a week before the trip, my husband found out he, too, needed to be out of town. Since neither of us could cancel our trips, we beat our brains trying to think of some options. Our closest relatives were over a thousand miles away and asking neighbors to pitch in for that long would be an imposition.

So, I tentatively gave Mom and Dad a call. They had both retired a few months earlier, but hadn't yet had time to do the things they had planned after raising nine children and working full-time. Although they pitched in with the other grandkids who lived nearby, it was never for more than a weekend. But I tried. "Mom, as you know I'm traveling next week in the Maryland/New Jersey area, just a few hours from where you live. Unfortunately, Lorin also needs to be out of town that week. I know it's a lot to ask, but I was wondering if I could bring Alexandra with me and have you and Dad drive down to Baltimore and spend the week traveling with us. We could all share a hotel room, you could take care of Alexandra until I finished work at 5pm, we could

187

all have dinner together, and then drive on to the next city where I'm speaking. I'd be most grateful, if you could help. Just this once. Please?"

Let's face it, that probably doesn't sound like that much fun. But you know Moms. She agreed, yet I could tell from her voice that (after all these years being states apart from each others) spending so much time cooped up with each other may not be easy.

But we all found out otherwise. First, I enjoyed my parents more when we were away from the rest of the clan. My daughter and my parents had a blast bonding together all day without Mom around – and they all got to see sights they'd never seen before. I was able to do my job and Alexandra got to see what I do when I'm on the road. My parents got to see more of the country for very little money. Although I was a bit leary in the beginning, I think bringing Alexandra along helped to strengthen my business relationships. And, most importantly, I got to spend time with Alexandra. My parents and I enjoyed traveling together so much and the arrangement has worked out well that we purposely plan trips together – about four a year! At the age of 10, Alexandra has already visited 30 states and eight countries!

So, don't always leave home alone – take your family (or even friends) along. According to a recent National Business Travel Monitor study, one out of every five business travelers took their children on at least one trip last year. Here are some options for spending time with your family on the road:

▶ **Have Them Join You For the Weekend.**
- **Save the company some money.** Companies often offer to pay for the weekend expenses if you'll agree to stay over on a Saturday since the airline ticket will be considerably less. (Or if you normally fly business class,

maybe you can buy two coach class tickets for the price of one.) In addition, hotels often offer special rates (sometimes half price) for a weekend stay. In addition to taking family, take advantage of the travels to meet up with friends and family all over the world.

- **Make it a mini-vacation.** Use your travels as a "scouting" mission to plan family weekend trips or a get away with your significant other. Then book business on Thursday, Friday, and Monday so your family can fly in for the weekend. That's why you collect frequent flyer miles, isn't it? For something they'll treasure forever, have your children keep a log of places they have visited and share a few lines in the journal about what they saw, something funny they want to remember, or a gift they got.

▶ **Take Them With You for the Whole Trip.**

- **Invite a caretaker along.** Can you think of someone you can invite to come along with your children? I know one speaker who takes her husband and children along on every driving trip! There's still plenty of time for you all to have some fun together.
- **Take advantage of conference care.** Many conferences are now offering "conference care" – on-site child care and youth programming. You might think about bringing just one child at a time to make them feel more special.
- **Take the family on vacation while you work.** If you're going to places that your family wouldn't have an opportunity to see otherwise, take advantage of it.
- **In the summer, many of the hotels have activities for children.** Although there are often age limits, activities include swimming, art lessons, games, and scavenger hunts. Most hotels offer kid-friendly menus. Ask them if they offer child-proof rooms and amenities such as cribs, high chairs, car seats, and strollers.
- **Hire a sitter.** Hotels can often arrange for an agency person or sitter. Talk to the concierge in advance and

189

ask for a bonded childcare agency. They'll usually charge $9-12 an hour.

▶ Put Them to Work.

- **Family can help you.** Invite your family along to help you in your business by returning phone calls or just acting as a personal valet. While doing some media spokesperson work, Alexandra was a big help when I only had one advertisement break to set up my props for television.

- **Encourage them to start a business.** There are many couples that travel together all the time. Although your partner could help you in their work, you could also encourage them to start a business (even part-time) that requires travel. Our friend's wife was a pretty good photographer. So she took a few photography courses and started taking stock photos to sell to the Chambers of the cities she visited with her husband.

Happy Travels!

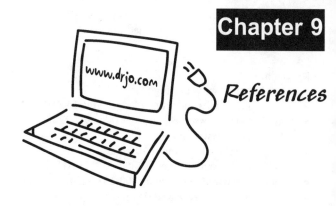

Chapter 9

References

In This Chapter:
▶Websites, books, and other invaluable information for the busy traveler

---

▶ **Accomodations:**

- **www.ase.net** – The Accomodation Search Engine for hotels, motels, and bed & breakfasts
- **www.bbonline.com** – Bed & Breakfast reservations
- **www.bedandbreakfast.com** – B&Bs reservations
- **www.bestwestern.com** – Best Western (800-528-1234)
- **www.daysinn.com** – Days Inn Hotels (800-325-2525)
- **www.doubletree.com** – DoubleTree (800-222-8733)
- **www.econolodge.com** – Econolodge Hotels
- **www.hilton.com** – Hilton Hotels (800-445-8667)
- **www.holiday-inn.com** – Holiday Inn (800-465-4329)
- **www.hyatt.com** – Hyatt Hotels (800-228-9000)
- **www.hotelguide.com** – lodging all over the world
- **www.marriot.com** – Marriot Hotels (800-228-9290)
- **www.radisson.com** – Radisson Hotels (800-333-3333)
- **www.starwood.com** – Sheraton (800-325-3535)

- **www.westin.com** – Westin Hotels (800-228-3000)
- **www.wyndham.com** – Wyndham (800-WYNDHAM)

▶ **Airlines:**

- Aer Lingus – **www.aerlingus.ie**
- Air Aruba – **www. interknowledge.com/air-aruba**
- Air Canada – **www.aircanada.ca** (888-247-2262)
- Air France – **www.airfrance.fr**
- Air New Zealand – **www.airnz.co.nz**
- AirTran – **www.airtran.com** (800-AIR-TRAN)
- Aloha – **www.alohaair.com** (800-367-5250)
- America West – **www.americanwest.com** (800-235-9292)
- American Airlines – **www.aa.com** (800-433-7300)
- Ansett Australia – **www.ansett.com.au**
- Asiana – **http://us.flyasiana.com**
- Australian – **www.aua.co.at/aua**
- Cathay Pacific – **www.cathay-usa.com**
- Continental – **www.flycontinental.com** (800-525-0280)
- Delta – **www.delta.com** (800-221-1212)
- El Al – **www.elal.co.il**
- Finnair – **www.finnair.fi**
- KLM UK – **www.klmuk.com** (800-374-7747)
- Lauda Air – **www.laudaair.com**
- Mexicana – **www.mexicana.com** (800-531-7921)
- Northwest – **www.nwa.com** (800-225-2525)
- Quantas – **www.quantas.com.au** (800-227-4500)
- Scandinavian – **www.sas.se** (800-221-2350)
- Southwest – **www.iflyswa.com** (800-435-9792)
- Swissair – **www.swissair.ch**
- Trans World – **www.twa.com** (800-221-2000)
- Transwede – **www.transwede.com**
- United – **www.ual.com** (800-241-6522)
- US Airways – **www. usair.com** (800-428-4322)
- Virgin Atlantic Airways – **www.fly.virgin.com**

▶ **Family Travel:**

- **www.familytravelforum.com** – Founded by business professionals with global family travel experience, this site (for a fee) offers unbiased information, informed advice and practical tips designed to make family traveling a rewarding, safe, and hassle-free experience.
- **www.familyonboard.com** – online catalog for CDs, tapes, guidebooks, and travel products for kids.
- **www.flyingwithkids.com** – Air travel advice and travel tips for families with pre-school age children.

▶ **Fitness:**

- **http://courseguide.golfweb.com** – search for a golf course at your destination.
- **http://lornet.com/SGOL** – Bill Haverland and Tom Saunders maintain a list of year round, public & private, swimming pools that admit for free or a day rate.
- **www.24hourfitness.com** – 24 Hour Fitness or Q Sports Club offers an All-Club membership that allow you to visit any of their locations in the US or abroad at no charge for up to 30 days.
- **www.americanhiking.org** – The only national organization dedicated to serving hikers and protecting the nation's hiking trails. Volunteer Vacations offer folks an opportunity to get away for 1-2 week service trips.
- **www.americanrunning.org** – The American Running Association offers running maps from all over the world.
- **www.collagevideo.com** – offers hundreds of exercise videos (800-433-6769).
- **www.fitforbusiness.com** – hotels that offer great fitness rooms, plus links to many fitness sites.
- **www.fitnesslink.com** – Information site offering free tips, recipes, and workouts to help you stay fit.
- **www.frogsonice.com/skateweb/clubs.html** – where to find an ice skating rink.

- **www.ihrsa.com** - The International Health, Racquet & Sportsclub Association (IHRSA) is a not-for-profit trade association representing health & fitness facilities. Their Passport Program grants reciprocal guest privileges in some over 3,500 IHRSA member health clubs in over 50 countries for a discount.
- **www.rollerskate.net** – find a roller skating rink in your city.
- **www.runnersworld.com/onthroad/home.html** – offers information on hotels with outstanding fitness clubs, running courses, and races all over the world.
- **www.sportsmatchonline.com** – helps travelers or newcomers connect with other sportminded individuals for running and matches.
- **www.sportsmusic.com** – music to fit your preferences and workout pace (800-878-4764).
- **www.spriproducts.com** – *Xertubes*® and other fitness equipment (800-222-7774).
- **www.squashtalk.com** – International travel directory of squash courts.

▶ **Health:**
- **www.apneanet.org** – information for people with apnea.
- **www.cdc.gov/travel** – health-related travel information for specific destinations including health recommendations, disease outbreaks, and required and recommended vaccines. Toll-free number is 877-FYI-TRIP. The toll-free fax number for requesting information is 888-232-3299.
- **www.cdc.gov/health/diseases.htm** – Information (symptoms, diagnosis, and treatment) on hundreds of diseases including those caused by viruses, parasites, worms, bacteria, and ameobas.
- **www.dininglean.com** – Dr Jo's website on how to eat healthy in your favorite restaurants. Includes information and links to her book, Dining Lean.

- **www.drweil.com** – Dr Weils's natural health site.
- **www.eatright.org** – The American Dietetic Association's web site offers "Find a Dietitian" services plus information on nutrition.
- **www.flyana.com** – airline passenger guide to safe, healthy air travel by former flight attendant Diana Fairechild. Tips on fear of flying.
- **www.hc-sc.gc.ca/hpb/lcdc** – Health Canada provides health information for Canadian travelers including health advisories and list of travel clinics across Canada.
- **www.healthfinder.gov** – health info from the Department of Health & Human services.
- **www.intellihealth.com** – medical info from John Hopkins.
- **www.mayohealth.org** – prescription index and medical encyclopedia.
- **www.navigator.tufts.edu** – ranks nutrition web sites.
- **www.northernlight-tech.com** – Northern Light Technologies sell bright lights that are helpful for persons suffering from Seasonal Affective Disorder (SAD) or jet lag.
- **www.vrg.org/travel** – The Vegetarian Resource Group offers tips for vegetarian business travelers, recommended resources, plus specific restaurant recommendations for selected US cities.
- **www.who.int** – Comprehensive health information from the World Health Organization including information on common diseases, vaccine requirements, and treatment regimes.
- **www.sleepfoundation.org** – The National Sleep Foundation offers info and tips on getting a good night's sleep.
- **www.webmd.com** – comprehensive health information.

▶ **Helpful Information for Travelers:**

- **300 Incredible Things for Travelers on the Internet** – Ken Leebow offers 300 websites of interest to travelers in this book. (www.300Incredible.com, 800-909-6505)

- **Do's and Taboos Around the World** – a book by Roger Axtell (1993).

- **Inside Flyer magazine** – this is the monthly guide to all the ways to earn frequent flyer miles and use them. If there's anything to do with your favorite frequent flyer, hotel and credit card program, it's in here – every month. (www.insideflyer.com or call 800-333-5937).

- **The Official Frequent Flyer Guidebook** – updated annually, this 600 page book has everything you've ever wanted to know about frequent flyer programs. From award charts to advice on managing your programs, this is the one book you don't fly without (www.insideflyer.com, 800-333-5937).

- **Travel Rights** – this helpful book by Charles Leocha describes how to get the best travel deals and get help with travel emergencies. In addition, he explains how to interpret the fine print in airline, rental car, and credit card company's rules and policies.

- **Ultimate Internet Travel Planning Guide** – listings and reviews of over 400 travel-related sites written by Lisa Weber (www.lisaweber.com) who speaks on communication, motivation, and traveling in the US and abroad (520-722-5455, toll-free 877-580-5455).

- **www.aaa.com** – AAA is a not-for-profit federation of 84 automobile clubs throughout the United States and Canada and the largest leisure travel agency in North America.

- **www.airporthub.com** – links to official sites of airports all over the world.

- **www.airsafe.com** – information about accidents and fatal events on specific aircraft and airlines, air rage, fear of flying, baggage information and more.

- **www.businesstravel.about.com** – hundreds of articles and discussions about business and recreational travel (including information for disabled travelers) plus links to travel sites.

- **www.customs.ustreas.gov** – US customs information. Traveler section includes information regarding entering and leaving the US, restricted/prohibited merchandise, medications/drugs, pets/animals, and mailing goods to the US.

- **www.faa.gov** – Airline safety and security violations, fines, and accidents reported by the US Federal Aviation Association, airport links.

- **www.fhwa.dot.gov/trafficinfo/index.htm** – The US Federal Highway Administration provides information and links to national traffic and road closure information plus real-time traffic maps for many major cities.

- **www.fmcsa.dot.gov** – Federal Motor Carrier Safety Administration resources for the nation's interstate commercial carrier industry.

- **www.flyertalk.com** – with almost 500,000 posts from frequent travelers sharing their best tips and information, it's the world's largest bulletin board devoted to travel and frequent flyer programs.

- **www.fbtc.com** – Frequent Business Traveler's Club.

- **www.iapa.com** – International Airline Passenger's Association.

- **www.myparkguide.com** – information on the US National Parks, including park use, activities, fees, maps and directions, and nearby attractions.

- **www.rulesoftheair.com** – Terry Trippler provides explanations to dozens of topics which the airlines detail in the Contract of Carriage accompanying each airline ticket purchase.

- **www.travel.state.gov** – The US State Department of Consular Affairs provides information including travel publications, travel warnings, consular information sheets, list of lawyers abroad, lists of doctor/hospitals abroad, and passport and visa information.

- **http://times.clari.net.au** – Find out what time it is all over the world.
- **www.usatoday.com** – Business travel news updated daily from USA Today.
- **www.worldtime.org** – info on local times all over the world, sunrise and sunset times, and public holidays.

▶ **Luggage, Clothes, and Accessories:**
- **www.briggs-riley.com** – luggage.
- **www.brookstoneonline.com** – unique and useful assessories for the traveler.
- **www.landsend.com** – clothing, luggage (800-356-4444).
- **www.llbean.com** – clothing, luggage, accessories (800-221-4221).
- **www.magellans.com** – clothing, accessories, and luggage (800-962-4943).
- **www.travelsmith.com** – accessories, clothing, luggage (800-950-1600).
- **www.rei.com** – clothing, backpacks, camping equipment, assessories for travelers.
- **www.safetravel.com** – travel emergency medical, dental, and blister fighter kits. Also includes links to travel health information and insurance.
- **www.sharperimage.com** – travel accessories, convenience items (800-344-4444).
- **www.swissarmy.com** – travel gear, briefcases, pocket knives, watches.
- **www.travelaccessories.com** – accessories.
- **www.travelproducts.com** – accessories (800-917-4616).
- **www.travelsupplies.com** – accessories.
- **www.traveltools.com** – accessories.
- **www.worldtraveler.com** – luggage and accessories.

▶ **Maps:**
- **www.mapblast.com** – includes ski lodging information.
- **www.mapquest.com**
- **www.maps.com**
- **www.mapstore.com**
- **www.randmcnally.com**
- **www.switchboard.com** – find a person, get maps and directions.

▶ **Money:**
- **www.mastercard.com** – ATM locator.
- **www.oanda.com** – Currency converter, daily (and historical) currency exchange rates, and foreign exchange tables for travelers, investors, and businesses.
- **www.visa.com** – ATM locator.
- **www.xe.net** – Currency converter

▶ **Passports:**
- **www.travel.state.gov/passport_services.html** – how and where to apply for a passport, change your name.
- **www.passportexpress.com** – claims to be able to send out passports 24 hours after they receive the materials. They charge a $100-150 fee in addition to government fees (401-272-4612).

▶ **Safety:**
- **http://travel.state.gov/travel_warnings.html** – US State Department of Consular Affairs maintains up-to-date travel warnings.
- **www.hc-sc.gc.ca/hpb/lcdc** – health information for Canadian travelers includes health advisories and list of travel clinics across Canada.
- **www.uma.org/usdotsaf.htm** – bus and motorcoach company safety records maintained by the US Department of Transportation's Office of Motor Carrier Safety.

▶ **Travel Bookings:**

In addition to travel information and reservations, most sites also provide (or have links to) car and hotel reservations, maps and driving directions, and weather information.

- **www.1travel.com**
- **www.11thhourvacations.com**
- **www.biztravel.com** –In addition to reservations, this site provides many links and helpful columns including "MileMaster" by Randy Petersen, "On the Road to Good Health" tips by Dr. Eliot Heher, "The Tactical Traveler" by road warrior Joe Brancatelli, and "The Travel Technologist" by Christopher Elliot.
- **www.cheaptickets.com**
- **www.cheapertravel.com** – Home of Pavlus Travel, largest reseller of Trafalgar and Insight Tours.
- **www.concierge.com** – includes many valuable links.
- **www.expedia.com**
- **www.Fodors.com** – includes tips for travelers, discussions of hotels and restaurants, and information on cruises and adventure travel.
- **www.flyaow.com** – Airline of the Web offers reservations, tips for travelers, and toll-free phone numbers for airlines.
- **www.Frommers.com** – Arthur Frommer's Budget Travel includes vacation ideas and packages.
- **www.hoovers.com** – this comprehensive source of business information includes a section under "Business Travel" with travel reservations, city guides, travel information, flight tracking information, connections to travel gear, and an online copy center.
- **www.ivillage.com/travel** – includes many travel tips.
- **www.lastminutetravel.com**
- **www.lowestfare.com**
- **www.mytravelguide.com**
- **www.onetravel.com**
- **www.qixo.com** – compares fares from many sites.

- www.site59.com
- **www.spectrav.com** – Specialty Travel Index has tours for adventure and special-interest vacations worldwide.
- **www.travel.com** – Travel services including rail passes, vacation packages, and tickets to the latest events.
- http://travel.yahoo.com
- www.Travelocity.com
- www.trip.com

▶ **Miscellaneous:**

- **www.jewishtravel.com** – Tips for kosher dining around the globe as well as kosher and non-kosher house exchange service.
- **www.petswelcome.com** – 25,000 listing of hotels, inns, and B&B that like your pet as much as you do plus tips on traveling or moving with pets.

▶ **Speaking the Language:**

- **www.berlitz.com** – products to teach you another language. Books include Berlitz European Menu Reader (pocket-sized book containing a 15 language glossary to help travelers know what they're ordering on the menu) and the Berlitz Business Travel Guide to Europe.
- **www.dailylinguist.com** – free daily eZine to learn a foreign language one phrase at a time, bookstore.
- **www.travlang.com** – offers on-line translating dictionaries, on-line and CD-ROM traveler's language courses.

How to Stay Healthy & Fit on the Road

▶ **Special Needs:**

- **www.access-able.com** – Access Able Travel Source offers tours, resources and travel tales for the hearing- or sight-impaired and the physically handicapped, plus a newsletter and links to relevant sites.
- **www.GimpontheGo.com** – tips and products for the disabled.

▶ **Technology:**

- **www.roadnews.com** – tips on traveling with laptops.
- **kropla.com** – help for travelers who want to make sure their laptops work anywhere. Features easy-to-read chart detailing voltage and plug type used in almost every country. World wide phone guide troubleshoots problems you're likely to hit hooking up your modem overseas.

▶ **Traveling Solo:**

- **www.cstn.org** – Connecting: Solo Travel Network provides tips, tales, and tours for people traveling alone.
- **www.solodining.com** – Marya Charles Alexander's newsletter and national directory of restaurants with communal tables is devoted to taking the bite out of eating alone (800-299-1079).

▶ **Weather:**

- **www.weather.com** – offers 10 day forecasts.
- **www.accuweather.com**
- **www.intellicast.com**
- **www.nws.noaaa.com** – National Weather Service.

▶ **What's Happening?**

Find out what's going on in the city of your destination:

- **www.bts.gov/virtualib** – Links to airlines, international mass transit, and cycling clubs.
- **www.citypass.net** – CityPass offers discounted booklet for admission tickets to attractions in Boston, Chicago, New York, Philadelphia, San Francisco, or Seattle.
- **www.citysearch.com** – make the most of your city.
- **www.guidebooks.com** – traveler guide books.
- **www.lonelyplanet.com** – guidebooks for travelers.
- **www.officialtravelinfo.com** – The International Association of Convention and Visitor's Bureaus offers links to bureaus all over the world.
- **www.ontheroad.com** – restaurants, entertainment, museums, galleries, business events, sports, and other tips for the city of your destination.
- **www.tourstates.com** – National Council of State Tourism links to attractions, events, and places in the US region of your choice.
- **www.towd.com** – lists only official government tourism offices, convention and visitors bureaus, chambers of commerce, and similar agencies which provide free, accurate, and unbiased travel information to the public.
- **www.ticketmaster.com** – buying tickets for shows etc.
- **www.usacitylink.com** – links to state and city information including vacation rentals, things to do, and other resources.

How to Stay Healthy & Fit on the Road

▶ **Women Travelers:**

- **www.womenbusinesstravelers.com** – great tips for women travelers from Wyndham Hotels & Resorts.
- **www.women-traveling.com** – escorted, small group travel for women.
- **www.journeywoman.com** – tips and newsletter for women travelers. Includes tips on culturally correct dining, what to wear in different cities around the world, and boards to meet other women travelers.

▶ **Your rights:**

- **www.passengerrights.com** – "makes it easy to complain when airlines, hotels, and the rest treat you just like another piece of cargo."
- **www.ticked.com** – tips for ticked off passengers.

Joanne V. Lichten, PhD, RD

helping busy people stay healthy & sane

Dr Jo's your ticket to staying healthy & sane in this whirlwind world. She's available to speak to your company, group, or association.

Call today: 1-888-431-5326

Topics include:

How to Stay Healthy & Fit (for travelers or busy people)

Defensive Dining (how to eat healthy in restaurants)

Keeping Your Energy Up All Day Long

Swimming in a Sea of Priorities
(stress management & life in balance)

How to Defuse Anger & Calm People Down

How to Fix an Attitude (dealing with negativity)

Dealing with Difficult People

Stay Calm, State Your Case, & Be Listened To

How to Enjoy the Ride of Your Life

Order Form

For credit card orders (Visa, MC, Discover)
or to inquire about quantity discounts
call 1-888-431-5326
or email nutrifitbooks@aol.com

_____ copies of *Dining Lean* @ \$14.95 each _____

_____ copies of *How to Stay Healthy*

     & Fit on the Road @ \$9.95 each _____

If shipping to Texas add 7¼% _____

Shipping cost (\$4/1book, \$1/each add'l) _____

Total _____

Name:_____

Address:_____

City:_____ State:_____ Zip:_____

Phone: _____ Email: _____

Send check or money order to:
Nutrifit Publishing
PO Box 690452
Houston, TX 77269-0452

Joanne V. Lichten, PhD, RD

helping busy people stay healthy & sane

Dr Jo's your ticket to staying healthy & sane in this whirlwind world. She's available to speak to your company, group, or association.

Call today: 1-888-431-5326

Topics include:

How to Stay Healthy & Fit (for travelers or busy people)

Defensive Dining (how to eat healthy in restaurants)

Keeping Your Energy Up All Day Long

Swimming in a Sea of Priorities
(stress management & life in balance)

How to Defuse Anger & Calm People Down

How to Fix an Attitude (dealing with negativity)

Dealing with Difficult People

Stay Calm, State Your Case, & Be Listened To

How to Enjoy the Ride of Your Life

Order Form

For credit card orders (Visa, MC, Discover)
or to inquire about quantity discounts
call 1-888-431-5326
or email nutrifitbooks@aol.com

_____ copies of *Dining Lean* @ $14.95 each _____

_____ copies of *How to Stay Healthy*

                & Fit on the Road @ $9.95 each _____

If shipping to Texas add 7¼% _____

Shipping cost ($4/1book, $1/each add'l) _____

Total _____

Name:_____

Address:_____

City:_____ State:_____ Zip:_____

Phone: _____ Email: _____

Send check or money order to:
Nutrifit Publishing
PO Box 690452
Houston, TX 77269-0452
